Praise for *The Seed of Intelligence*

Believe it or not, everything starts in the womb. A pregnancy's full potential can be reached through a careful analysis and adjustment of the mother's external and mental world... "*Your Baby's Developing Brain*" Series by Dr. Chong Chen is a great resource to add to your knowledge about the way we function as humans and how to assist future tiny humans to reach their best physical and psychological potential.

— **Lucia Grosaru**, Psychology Corner

A groundbreaking synthesis of the state-of-the-art scientific data, *The Seed of Intelligence* is a great resource for all expecting parents.

— **Yutaka Matsuoka**, M.D., Ph.D.
Chief, Division of Health Care Research,
Center for Public Health Sciences
National Cancer Center Japan
Vice President, International Society for Nutritional
Psychiatry Research

Your Baby's Developing Brain Series II

THE SEED OF INTELLIGENCE

Boost Your Baby's Developing Brain through Optimal Nutrition and Healthy Lifestyle

CHONG CHEN, PH.D.

Brain & Life Publishing

London

ISBN 978-1-9997601-3-7 E-book

ISBN 978-1-9997601-4-4 Paperback

Brain & Life Publishing

27 Old Gloucester Street, London, U.K.

Printed in the United Kingdom. First Printing, 2017

For information about special needs for bulk purchases, sales promotions, and educational needs, please contact orders@brainandlife.net.

ALSO BY CHONG CHEN

Plato's Insight: How Physical Exercise Boosts Mental Excellence

Fitness Powered Brains: Optimize Your Productivity, Leadership and Performance

Psychology for Pregnancy: How Your Mental Health during Pregnancy Programs Your Baby's Developing Brain (Your Baby's Developing Brain Series I)

Our old notion of nature influencing the fetus before birth and nurture after birth needs an update. There is an antenatal environment, too, that is provided by the mother.

Psychologist Janet DiPietro
Johns Hopkins University

To my parents for their love and support

Table of Contents

PREFACE 1

PART 1: THE SEED OF INTELLIGENCE 3

1. Your baby experiences a remarkable rate of development in the womb 4

2. The seed of intelligence dissected 6

3. Pregnancy provides a perfect opportunity for health revolution 9

4. Many people make changes during pregnancy, but most lack adequate knowledge on a healthy lifestyle 10

5. Why is unplanned pregnancy dangerous? 13

6. Concerns for single mothers 15

7. I'm giving birth in rapid succession or to twins, what should I be wary of? 17

8. How often should I attend antenatal care during pregnancy? 18

PART 2: DIET & NUTRITION 21

9. How does maternal undernutrition affect the baby? Lessons from the 1944–1945 Dutch Famine and the 1959–1961 Chinese Famine 22

10. What if I'm very thin? 24

11. Can I diet while pregnant? 26

12. Why shouldn't I skip meals? 28

13. Are vegan-vegetarian diets dangerous during pregnancy? 29

14. How much extra energy intake do I need? 30

15. What is the most recommended healthy diet?..................33

16. Why should I eat fruits and vegetables daily?..................36

17. How much fruit should I eat daily?..................38

18. How many vegetables should I eat daily?..........................39

19. How much and what kind of protein should I consume daily?..40

20. Why should I eat seafood regularly?................................42

21. Seafood may be contaminated by mercury, should I still eat it frequently? 43

22. Can I eat canned seafood?..45

23. How much and what kind of seafood should I eat per week? 46

24. Why should I consume dairy?..47

25. How much and what kind of dairy should I consume every day?..48

26. What is the consequence of a "western" diet? 49

27. What is the consequence of a high-fat diet?......................51

28. Is being obese bad for me?...52

29. Is being obese bad for my baby?......................................54

30. How much gestational weight gain is healthy and why? ..56

31. How can I deal with obesity and prevent excessive weight gain during pregnancy? 58

32. What foods help deal with stress and prevent depression?..60

33. How to successfully start a healthy diet change?..............61

34. What is mindful eating and why is it important? 62

PART 3: NUTRITION SUPPLEMENTATION 65

   35. What supplements should I take during pregnancy and
       why? 66

   36. Introduction to nutrients (1): Folic acid 68

   37. Introduction to nutrients (2): Iron 70

   38. Introduction to nutrients (3): Vitamin D 73

   39. Introduction to nutrients (4): Multiple micronutrient
       supplements 75

   40. Introduction to nutrients (5): Omega-3 PUFA 79

   41. Introduction to nutrients (6): The ratio of omega-6 to
       omega-3 PUFA 82

PART 4: FOOD SAFETY & SUBSTANCE ABUSE 85

   42. Can I drink coffee and tea during pregnancy? 86

   43. Why should I stop eating fried potato chips and
       cookies? 88

   44. How can soft cheese, raw sprouts, and melons be
       dangerous? 89

   45. How dangerous is smoking for me? 92

   46. Does smoking affect my baby? 94

   47. Should family members stop smoking during
       pregnancy? 97

   48. Why should I avoid any alcohol? 98

   49. Toxic chemicals (1): Cocaine 99

   50. Toxic chemicals (2): Cannabis 100

   51. Toxic chemicals (3): Methamphetamine 101

**PART 5: WORK, PHYSICAL EXERCISE, &
ENVIRONMENTAL RISKS** 103

52. Does my job affect my baby? 104

53. Why should I live and work in a quiet, non-noisy
    place? 106

54. Should I stop shiftwork during pregnancy? 108

55. Is physical exercise recommended during pregnancy? ...110

56. What are the benefits of utilizing green environments? ..112

57. Does air pollution affect me? 114

58. Does air pollution affect my baby? 115

59. Toxic chemicals (4): Lead 117

PART 6: SLEEP 119

60. What are the typical sleep problems during pregnancy? .120

61. How much sleep is necessary? 121

62. How does insufficient and poor sleep affect me? 122

63. Does my sleep affect my baby? 123

64. What if I snore? 124

65. Am I sleeping well? 125

66. How can I improve sleep quality? 126

POSTSCRIPT 129

REFERENCES 131

INDEX 201

ABOUT THE AUTHOR 205

PREFACE

This series was originally written for my family and friends. Given my training in medicine, psychiatry, and brain science, they had long been asking me what science says about pregnancy and parenting. For instance, how does one boost a baby's brain development? How can one raise a genius? Is there anything parents can do during pregnancy to ensure a healthy, intelligent, and happy child? To answer their questions, I decided to do extensive research myself. After all, I am a scientist. Now, after over six years of research, I have finally completed this comprehensive report.

My primary interest lies in brain development. There are already many popular books on how to promote the physical health of babies but brain development, in contrast, is only a recent scientific topic. Our brain determines our intellectual, emotional, and social functioning. The latter defines who we are. As Rene Descartes put it, "I think, therefore I am." That's it.

I have gone through all the necessary medical training in gynaecology (the medical field dealing with female reproductive systems), obstetrics (pregnancy and childbirth) and pediatrics (the care of infants and children). Yet, I myself was astonished by the results of my research. Parents' health and behaviors, which may seem subtle to themselves, exert a powerful and lost-lasting impact on their infant's developing brain and some of that impact persists well into adulthood. Consequently, I feel that the results of my research should be available to every parent.

Then came this series, which I'd like to call "*Your Baby's Developing Brain*." The first three volumes of this series focus on the period of pregnancy. They are about what parents can do during pregnancy to protect and boost their baby's developing brain. The first volume focuses on the psychological health of the parents during pregnancy, and is entitled *Psychology for Pregnancy: How Your Mental Health during Pregnancy Programs Your Baby's Developing Brain*. The second volume, namely the present book, introduces a healthy maternal lifestyle, including proper nutrition and sleep, etc. The third volume focuses on antenatal education or *taijiao*, i.e., educating babies in the womb. I have planned more volumes on postpartum parenting. If you want to get a notification when a new volume is released, please sign up for my newsletter at https://brainandlife.net.

PART 1: THE SEED OF INTELLIGENCE

1. Your baby experiences a remarkable rate of development in the womb

The formation of a zygote marks the beginning of the new life of your baby. It then undergoes three distinct stages:

1) *The pre-embryonic stage*, or the first two weeks: a period of cell division and differentiation;

2) *The embryonic period*, or from week 3 to 8: a period of the formation of tissues and organs;

3) *The fetal period*, or from week 9 until birth: a period of the maturation of tissues and organs and rapid growth of the body and brain.

During gestation, your baby experiences an extremely rapid development, particularly in the brain and nervous system, which is unmatched at any other stage in life.

Neurogenesis, namely the creation of new neurons, initiates on embryonic day 42 and finishes by midgestation. During this period, neurogenesis can occur at a remarkable rate of over 100,000 new cells per minute. These new cells migrate and form synapses (or synaptic connections) and communicate with each other. Synapses are the substrate of memory and other cognitive processes. During the third trimester (from week 28 to birth), it is estimated that per minute around 40,000 synapses can be formed.

The fast development of the fetal brain renders the fetus susceptible to various influences by you, the mother. As we have discussed in *Psychology for Pregnancy*, your physical and psychological states determine your baby's growth environment. On one hand, accompanying the rapid development of the fetus the nutritional requirement increases. This can only be fulfilled by the mother's intake. Your nutrition is your baby's nutrition. On the other hand, you produce numerous chemicals in your body, good and bad, which are dependent on your lifestyle, including sleep habits, physical exercise, and work. These chemicals cross the placenta and exert powerful and lost-lasting impacts on your baby's developing brain.

Given an enriched, nourishing, and stimulating environment such as optimal nutrition and a healthy lifestyle, your baby will thrive. Given an impoverished, stressful, and toxic environment such as poor nutrition and an unhealthy lifestyle, your baby will wither. Therefore, an enriched environment is the seed of your baby's developing brain, his or her levels of intelligence and mental health. And your nutritional status and lifestyle during pregnancy determine the seed.

2. The seed of intelligence dissected

If we dissect an enriched environment from a neurobiological perspective, four pillars are at the core of its components.

The first pillar is a well-balanced nutritional supply, which provides all the necessary macronutrients and micronutrients, and satisfies the requirements of the mother and fetus. As we will see later, nutrients are the building blocks of our lives especially our brains.

The second pillar is an increased maternal blood level of neurotrophin factors particularly the brain-derived neurotrophic factor (BDNF). The maternal blood level of BDNF corresponds with that of the fetal brain and BDNF supports the production, growth, differentiation, and survival of neurons.

The third pillar is a reduced maternal level of the stress hormone cortisol. Exposure to continuously increasing levels of cortisol damages the brain and causes many physical and psychological problems in both the mother and the unborn child.

The fourth pillar is a lower maternal level of systemic inflammation, namely lower circulating level of pro-inflammatory cytokines. Pro-inflammatory cytokines are excreted from immune-related cells upon activation of the immune system because of infection, psychological stress or unhealthy lifestyles. Inflammation inhibits neurogenesis (the production of new neurons), impairs neurotransmission (the communication between neurons, which is the substrate of all cognitive processes), and induces cognitive deficits, sickness, and depression. Chronically high levels of maternal inflammation are toxic to both the mother and the fetus. It has been associated with an increased risk of maternal hypertension, poor placental functioning, fetus growth restriction, preterm birth, and low birth weight.

These four pillars are inter-correlated, each influences the rest. For instance, a healthy diet with a well-balanced nutrition increases blood levels of BDNF while reducing that of cortisol and systemic inflammation. Optimal maternal nutrition and a healthy lifestyle will promote these four pillars and lead to optimal physical and mental outcomes in the mother and her offspring. These outcomes are not only beneficial during pregnancy, but also years later.

(Actually, in any individual of any age from children to the elderly, a healthy lifestyle that promotes these four pillars will enhance one's physical and mental development, and improve achievement at school and work. And most, if not all, self-help books on health and diet are written surrounding activities related to these four pillars. Therefore, the seed of intelligence for your baby is also the seed of intelligence for you and your family. Pregnancy provides an opportunity for you to learn essential knowledge now that has life-long benefits.)

3. Pregnancy provides a perfect opportunity for health revolution

First, pregnancy typically occurs in early adulthood, at a time when most women are still forming their dietary habits and other lifestyle choices.

Second, the early stage of marriage or cohabitation is often when women adjust their food intake to that of their partners (and vice versa).

Third, women are the gatekeepers of the family diet. Even today, women are more likely to plan, buy, and prepare food at home than men.

Fourth, pregnancy is a time of increased nutritional requirements. During pregnancy, women must "eat for two" (see item 14), as the nutrients essential for healthy development of the fetus are completely determined by the mother.

Fifth, the mother's eating habits, even those during pregnancy (see item 16), affect the offspring's food preferences.

Your health and nutritional awareness have a substantial influence on the whole family's future health. Pregnancy provides a perfect time frame to learn sufficient knowledge and achieve a health revolution, with life-long benefits for the whole family.

4. Many people make changes during pregnancy, but most lack adequate knowledge on a healthy lifestyle

There's no doubt that, for most people, bringing a new life into the world is the greatest joy they will experience, and is one of the most challenging things they will face. More people come to realize that a healthy maternal lifestyle, including an adequate diet, is vital for the development of their baby's brain.

To safeguard their unborn child, many (but not all) people make lifestyle changes during pregnancy. For instance, research shows that the vast majority of women increase energy intake during pregnancy. They also increase intake of vegetables and fruits, while decreasing smoking and the consumption of fried and fast food, alcohol, caffeine-containing and sugar-sweetened drinks.

But despite these positive changes, the vast majority of pregnant women still fail to meet the recommendations of food and nutrient intake and levels of physical exercise by national and international guidelines. In a 2009 Australian study, merely 9% of the pregnant mothers met the recommendations of four servings of fruit per day, whereas only one-third met the recommendation of 30 minutes or more of moderate exercise on most days of the week. Two American cohort studies estimated that half to two-thirds of women who smoked cigarettes before pregnancy continued to smoke during pregnancy. According to a 2013 Greek study, passive smoking (second-hand smoking) in the household stayed unchanged, at a high rate of almost 60%. Finally, in a 2009 Hungarian study, over one-third of pregnant women drank at least one cup of coffee per day.

The reason why so many women (and their families) still keep an unhealthy lifestyle during pregnancy is simple: most people possess insufficient knowledge regarding what constitutes adequate nutrient intake and a healthy lifestyle during pregnancy and how this would affect their unborn child. In a 2013 Australian study, only 8% of pregnant women knew the correct recommended daily number of fruit servings (do you know this yourself?); more than half of them did not receive appropriate advice regarding healthy eating and physical exercise at the beginning of their pregnancy.

A 2011 study conducted in Tokyo showed that 69% of pregnant women believed that small babies would help a smooth delivery, whereas 36% were dieting during pregnancy. Among the dieters, 80% were based on self-judgment without consulting a dietician or doctor. It is true that small babies may help with a smooth delivery; however, small babies with low birth weight (birth weight less than 2500 grams) are at high risk of delayed physical and mental development. As we will see later, undernutrition because of maternal underweight and poor diet pose substantial risks to the healthy development of the fetus.

5. Why is unplanned pregnancy dangerous?

After conception, the zygote experiences the most rapid and revolutionary development. As we have mentioned, the first two weeks is a period of cell division and differentiation, the third to eighth week is a period of the formation of tissues and organs, whereas the production of neurons initiates on embryonic day 42. Therefore, this very beginning of the pregnancy is also the most susceptible period. With poor maternal nutrition and an unhealthy lifestyle, including smoking and drinking alcohol, the fetus may be negatively affected.

Furthermore, the greatest risk for most birth defects, including neural tube defects occurs during this period. Neural tube is the embryo's precursor to the central nervous system and neural tube defect is the incomplete close of the neural tube, which brings permanent nerve damage and causes stillbirths, neonatal death, or paralysis of the legs. To prevent neural tube defects, it has become common practice that all pregnant mothers take daily folic acid supplementation starting at least two months before pregnancy.

The reality is that almost half of pregnancies are unplanned, which subjects the fetus to substantial developmental risks.

Fortunately, research shows that daily multiple micronutrient supplementation during pregnancy (see item 39) can partly buffer or rescue the detrimental effects of prenatal alcohol exposure prior to pregnancy recognition.

If your pregnancy is unplanned, you should take recommended supplements (see Part 3 Nutrition Supplementation) and make lifestyle changes (see Part 2 Diet & Nutrition) immediately upon recognition of the pregnancy. You cannot change the past, but you can surely compensate for it and reduce any future risks.

6. Concerns for single mothers

In *Psychology for Pregnancy*, we discussed how married people are healthier and happier than unmarried people and that partner support is critical for physical and psychological health. Thus, single motherhood constitutes a risk for both the mother and fetus.

For single mothers, those living alone seem to have a higher risk than those living with parents. At least some of the increased risk can be attributed to the unhealthy diet of single mothers. For instance, single mothers have:

- Lower intakes of fruits and vegetables

- Higher intake of high-fat foods

- Higher intake of added sugar (sugar-sweetened beverages)

- More frequent smoking habits

The reason for this unhealthy diet may include financial insecurity, and feelings of stress and loneliness. As we have noted in *Psychology for Pregnancy*, stress and loneliness are detrimental to the fetus and can cause an unhealthy maternal diet. Therefore, if you are a single mother, pay careful attention to what you eat and adhere to a healthy diet. Living with parents, having supportive friends, attending pregnancy clubs, and other psychological strategies such as those of positive psychology and meditation (for more detailed introduction, see *Psychology for Pregnancy*) should be helpful.

7. I'm giving birth in rapid succession or to twins, what should I be wary of?

It has been shown that the maternal blood level of docosahexaenoic acid (DHA) reduces following each pregnancy and that, compared to those who have given birth once, mothers who have given birth in rapid succession and those who have given birth to twins or multiples have lower blood levels of DHA. Furthermore, the infant blood level of DHA also decreases as the number of infants per pregnancy increases. This also applies as the number of children the mother has given birth to increases.

As will be discussed in more detail below, DHA is an omega-3 polyunsaturated fatty acid (PUFA), which is essential for optimal brain development. The reduced maternal DHA restricts the growth of the fetus. The reduced infant DHA further inhibits the healthy development of the infant after birth.

Therefore, if you are giving birth in rapid succession (e.g., within one year of your previous delivery), or giving birth to twins or multiples, pay close attention to your diet and take omega-3 PUFA supplements (see item 40) in order to maintain an optimal status of nutritional supply to your baby.

8. How often should I attend antenatal care during pregnancy?

Antenatal care provides an opportunity for pregnant women to receive necessary examinations in order to prevent and treat potential health problems, and to get appropriate advice and information on a healthy pregnancy, childbirth, and postnatal recovery.

The World Health Organization (WHO) originally recommended pregnant women have at least four antenatal care assessments by or under the supervision of a healthcare professional. These should be spaced at regular intervals throughout pregnancy, starting as early as possible in the first trimester. At each antenatal care visit, the following routine care is offered to all pregnant women and babies:

- Confirmation of pregnancy

- Monitoring of progress of pregnancy and assessment of maternal and fetal well-being

- Detection of problems complicating pregnancy (e.g., anemia, hypertensive disorders, bleeding, malpresentations, multiple pregnancy)

- Respond to other reported complaints

- Tetanus immunization, anemia prevention and control (iron and folic acid supplementation)

- Information and counselling on self-care at home, nutrition, safer sex, breastfeeding, family planning, healthy lifestyle

- Birth planning, advice on danger signs and emergency preparedness

- Recording and reporting

- Syphilis testing

Research has shown that less than four antenatal visits are associated with a 6.8 times higher risk of low birth weight.

In the new 2016 *WHO Recommendations on Antenatal Care for a Positive Pregnancy Experience*, WHO recommends that the original four antenatal visits should be increased to eight, which are scheduled:

One visit during the first trimester (the first 12 weeks of pregnancy)

- Visit 1: up to 12 weeks

Two visits during the second trimester (from week 13 to 27 of pregnancy)

- Visit 2: 20 weeks

- Visit 3: 26 weeks

Five visits during the third trimester (from week 28 to birth)

- Visit 4: 30 weeks

- Visit 5: 34 weeks

- Visit 6: 36 weeks

- Visit 7: 38 weeks

- Visit 8: 40 weeks (Return for delivery at 41 weeks if not given birth)

This increased contact with a healthcare professional not only helps to detect problems earlier, but also helps pregnant mothers feel more secure and confident. It has been associated with a more positive pregnancy experience, including higher maternal satisfaction and lower perinatal mortality.

PART 2: DIET & NUTRITION

9. How does maternal undernutrition affect the baby? Lessons from the 1944–1945 Dutch Famine and the 1959–1961 Chinese Famine

Two tragic historical disasters provided valuable teaching lessons for prenatal undernutrition.

During the winter of 1944–1945 near the end of the Second World War, the German-occupied Western Netherlands was affected by an acute famine, known as the Hunger Winter. A German blockade cut off food supplies from farm areas and all the population, including pregnant women, received less than a quarter of the required calorie intake per day. It was found that women exposed to the famine during mid- to late gestation gave birth to babies with significantly reduced birth weights. Those exposed during early gestation gave birth to babies with normal weights, but who grew up to have higher rates of obesity. Furthermore, whereas babies exposed to the famine in utero during the first trimester were more likely to develop an addictive disorder and show lower executive function (a critical component of fluid intelligence) in adulthood, those exposed during the second or third trimester were more likely to develop a major affective disorder. Finally, regardless of the exposure time, all babies had a smaller adult head circumference, which suggests a smaller and less effective brain.

The 1959–1961 Chinese famine, or the Three Years of Great Chinese Famine, was another serious disaster. Prenatal exposure to this famine was associated with reduced executive function and increased risk of schizophrenia in adulthood.

These two tragic famines emphasize the importance of an adequate energy and nutrition intake during pregnancy.

10. What if I'm very thin?

A BMI of less than 18.5 is underweight, which suggests undernutrition. Your BMI is calculated as your weight in kilograms divided by the square of your height in meters. The prevalence of maternal underweight ranges from 10% to 19% in many counties. Sometimes undernutrition is a result of inflammatory processes, such as HIV or tuberculosis infection, which causes significant weight loss.

Maternal underweight has been associated with:

- Intrauterine growth restriction (which indicates a high developmental risk and is associated with cerebral palsy, cognitive deficits, behavioral problems, cardiovascular disease, type 2 diabetes, and stroke)

- A 1.24 times higher risk of spontaneous abortion

- A 1.29 times higher risk of preterm birth

- A 1.64 times higher risk of low birth weight

- Decreased language abilities at 12 months of age in the offspring

- Delayed cognitive development at 24 months of age in the offspring

If you are underweight, you had better pay serious attention to your diet and, by adhering to a balanced healthy diet, you can achieve the targeted weight gain during pregnancy (see item 30).

11. Can I diet while pregnant?

Better not, even you are overweight or obese.

Dieting during pregnancy will lead to insufficient energy and nutritional intake which fails the requirement of the developing fetus. Overweight and obesity pose great risk to the fetus (see item 29), but dieting is more risky.

According to a study conducted by Jesse S. Rodriguez at the University of Texas, compared to the offspring of baboons fed normal diets throughout gestation and lactation, offspring of baboons fed only 70% of food showed lower motivation (efforts towards getting rewards) and impaired working memory (a component of executive function essential for fluid intelligence) at three years of age. In another study with rats performed by the same author, 50% maternal protein restriction increased anxiety-like behaviors and the levels of stress hormone cortisol in the offspring.

Also, even among women with normal weight, many restrict their food intake during pregnancy to keep thin, or to have smaller infants, on the premise that smaller infants will carry a lower risk of delivery complications. However, infants who are small or disproportionate at birth have a high risk of delayed physical and mental development. They are more likely to die, get various infections, be shorter at adulthood, have lower cognitive ability, achieve less at school, have lower income, and develop diabetes, cancers, and mental health problems.

12. Why shouldn't I skip meals?

As mentioned above, maternal caloric/nutrition restriction is detrimental to the developing fetus. Skipping meals is a typical example of caloric/nutrition restriction. The U.S. National Academy of Medicine (previously Institute of Medicine) recommends that pregnant women should "eat small to moderate-sized meals at regular intervals, and eat nutritious snacks" to meet the developmental needs of the fetus.

Those who eat fewer than three meals (breakfast, lunch, and dinner) and two snacks (preferably fruits, vegetables, and dairy foods) per day have been estimated to be at a 1.30 times increased risk of preterm birth.

13. Are vegan-vegetarian diets dangerous during pregnancy?

Vegan-vegetarian women are more likely to be at risk of vitamin B12, iron, folate, zinc deficiencies, and tend to have lower blood levels of omega-3 PUFA DHA and eicosapentaenoic acid (EPA), which are essential for healthy development of the fetal brain. Therefore, vegan-vegetarian women should choose reliable food sources full of these nutrients (see below) or use supplements to meet the developmental requirement of the fetus.

14. How much extra energy intake do I need?

We mentioned that during pregnancy you should "eat for two." However, that literally means more nutritional than quantitative. In other words, you need a more balanced nutritional intake rather than excessive energy intake. The increase in energy intake during pregnancy is actually only moderate.

The U.S. Institute of Medicine (2006) recommends that:

- The first trimester (the first 12 weeks): no additional energy intake is needed.

- The second trimester (week 13–27): additional 340 kcal/day is needed.

- The third trimester (week 28 to birth): additional 452 kcal/day is needed.

Meanwhile, the U.K. National Institute for Health and Care Excellence (2010) recommends that no additional energy intake is needed in the first 6 months of pregnancy, while a slight increase of 200 kcal/day is needed in the final 3 months.

Examples of food or snack containing 200 kcal include:

- Almonds: 35g

- Peaches, dried, uncooked: 84g

- Salmon, Atlantic, wild, cooked: 110g

- Avocado: 125g

- Soybeans, green, cooked: 142g

- Fruit yogurt, low-fat: 190g

- Banana: 225g

- Plain yogurt, low-fat: 317g

- Apple, with skin: 385g

- Orange: 408g

- Low-fat milk (1%): 476g

Minister of Health Canada (2009) recommends that the extra energy intake can be achieved by an extra 2 to 3 snack or food servings each day, for instance:

- Have an extra morning snack of fruit with yogurt and an extra serving of vegetables with supper

- Have an extra glass of milk with lunch and supper

- Have an extra afternoon or evening snack of whole grain cereal with milk and sliced fruit or chopped nuts

- Have an extra afternoon snack of half a sandwich or whole grain toast with nut butter and a small glass of 100% orange juice

- Have an extra afternoon snack of dry meat or fish and a small piece of bannock

15. What is the most recommended healthy diet?

The Mediterranean-style diet is by far the most recommended healthy diet by the scientific community. The Mediterranean-style diet refers to the traditional dietary practices of countries bordering the Mediterranean Sea. It is characterized by:

1) High intake of plant foods: vegetables, fruits, legumes, and cereals

2) High intake of olive oil as the principal source of monounsaturated fat, but low intake of saturated fat such as butter

3) Moderate intake of fish

4) Low to moderate consumption of dairy products

5) Low consumption of meat and poultry

In the original Mediterranean-style diet, wine is consumed in low to moderate amounts. However, during pregnancy alcohol should be completely avoided (see item 48).

The Mediterranean-style diet promotes the four pillars of an enriched environment (see item 2). First, a Mediterranean-style diet is based on the regular intake of fruits and vegetables, lean choices of protein, omega-3 PUFA in the form of fatty fish, whole grains, and monounsaturated fatty acid from plant oils. It is nutritionally rich and well-balanced.

Second, a Mediterranean-style diet consumes fatty fish regularly. There are abundant omega-3 PUFA contained in fatty fish, which increases the level of BDNF in the maternal body;

Third, fatty fish contains abundant omega-3 PUFA, which helps to buffer psychological stress and reduces the release of cortisol (see item 32).

Fourth, polyphenols contained in vegetables and fruits and omega-3 PUFA in fatty fish are anti-inflammatory. High adherence to the Mediterranean-style diet has been associated with reduced blood concentrations of inflammation markers.

Thus, high adherence to the Mediterranean-style diet is associated with lower risk of maternal obesity, hypertension, diabetes, lower levels of psychological stress, depressive and anxious symptoms, and lower risk of preterm birth.

By far two large-scale cohort studies have examined the benefits of the Mediterranean-style diet during pregnancy, the Generation R Study which involved 8,879 pregnant women and their infants in Rotterdam, the Netherlands and the Norwegian Mother and Child Cohort Study which involved 23,020 pregnant women and their children in Norway. According to these two studies, high adherence to the Mediterranean-style diet during pregnancy was associated with less child externalizing problems (e.g., aggressive behaviors, attention deficit hyperactivity disorder or ADHD) and/or internalizing problems (depression, anxiety) during 1.5–6 years of age.

These positive outcomes are from research treating the Mediterranean-style diet as a pattern. The positive outcomes will be broader and more substantial if we examine each component of the diet independently.

One point that we have to be aware of is that although in the Mediterranean-style diet, dairy foods are consumed in only low to moderate amounts, research nevertheless shows that high intake of dairy foods bring many health benefits (see item 24 and 25).

16. Why should I eat fruits and vegetables daily?

Fruits and vegetables contain abundant polyphenols, which are anti-inflammatory. They also contain many key nutrients such as folate, magnesium, vitamin C, potassium, and other health-promoting non-essential compounds such as fiber. Furthermore, consumption of fruits and vegetables generally reduces the intake of other less nutrient-rich and junk foods.

In adults, high consumption of fruits and vegetables is associated with high cognitive function and low risk of chronic diseases such as cardiovascular disease and cancer.

During pregnancy, maternal consumption of fruits and vegetables has at least two benefits for the infant. First, it directly promotes the healthy development of the infant in the womb. A Canadian birth cohort study by Francois V. Bolduc at the University of Alberta showed that:

Each additional maternal daily serving of fruits (in the form of whole fruit or 100% fruit juice) consumed during pregnancy was associated with a significant improvement in the cognitive development of the infant at 1 year of age.

Second, maternal consumption of fruits and vegetables alters the flavor of her amniotic fluid, which changes the flavor preferences of her fetus (this is known as fetal learning, see Volume 3 of this series). After delivery, maternal consumption of fruits and vegetables alters the flavor of her milk, which similarly changes the flavor preferences of her infant. Therefore, maternal consumption of fruits and vegetables helps the infant to establish a life-long habit of a healthy diet. As shown by the Avon Longitudinal Study of Parents and Children which involved over 14,500 pregnancies in the Bristol area of U.K.:

Children whose mothers consumed more fruits and vegetables during pregnancy were more likely to eat fruits and vegetables at 2–4 years of age.

17. How much fruit should I eat daily?

The U.S. Department of Agriculture and Department of Health and Human Services recommend 2 cups (3–4 servings) of fruit per day for women at reproductive age. One cup of fruit can be either one cup of whole fruit or 100% fruit juice (about 8 oz. or 237 ml). Whole fruit includes raw, cooked, canned, frozen, and dried. The following amount is counted as one cup of fruit:

- One small apple about 6 cm in diameter

- A large peach of 7 cm in diameter

- A large orange of 7.5 cm in diameter

- A medium grapefruit of 10 cm in diameter

- A large banana about 20 cm long

- 8 large strawberries

- 14 grapes

Canadian scientist Francois V. Bolduc at the University of Alberta suggests that daily 3 cups (6–7 servings) of fruit may bring more benefits to the fetus's cognitive development.

18. How many vegetables should I eat daily?

The U.S. Department of Agriculture and Department of Health and Human Services recommend 2.5 cups (4–5 servings) of vegetables per day for women at reproductive age. This should include vegetables of different types and colors such as dark green (broccoli, spinach, leafy salad greens), red and orange (tomatoes, carrots, pumpkins), legumes (beans and peas), and starchy (potatoes, corn, cassava). This can be taken in all raw, cooked, frozen, canned, and dried forms, including vegetable juices. For instance, the following amount is counted as one cup of vegetables:

- One large green or red pepper about 8 cm in diameter

- One large tomato about 8 cm in diameter

- One large ear of corn about 20 cm long

- 2 medium carrots

- 2 large stalks of celery about 30 cm long

- 3 spears of broccoli about 13 cm long

Notably, in the case of raw leafy greens, 2 cups of raw leafy greens are considered equal to 1 cup of raw or cooked vegetables or vegetable juice.

19. How much and what kind of protein should I consume daily?

Every cell in our body and brain contains protein. Proteins are necessary for making enzymes, hormones, and neurotransmitters.

A healthy intake of protein includes a variety of protein foods from both animal and plant sources, including seafood, lean meats and poultry, eggs, legumes (beans and peas), nuts, seeds, and soy products.

The recommended amount of protein food consumed per day is 5.5 ounces (about 156 gram) equivalents of protein food. The following amount of food is considered as 1 ounce-equivalent of protein food:

- 1 ounce (28 gram) of cooked meat (lean beef, pork, or ham), poultry (chicken or turkey, without skin) or fish (e.g., salmon, trout, sardines)

- 1/4 cup cooked beans

- 1/4 cup (about 2 ounces, 28 gram) of tofu

- 1 egg

- 1 tablespoon of peanut butter

- 1/2 ounce (14 gram) of nuts or seeds (e.g., 12 almonds, 24 pistachios, 7 walnut halves)

Note that protein foods are rich in nutrients in addition to protein, including B vitamins, vitamin D, E, iron, omega-3 PUFA, selenium, choline, copper, zinc, and phosphorus, etc.

As seafood provides almost all of the omega-3 PUFA, to achieve a balanced diet, it is specifically recommended to eat seafood regularly (see item 20).

20. Why should I eat seafood regularly?

Coldwater, fatty fish such as salmon, herring, and sardines is rich in omega-3 PUFA and vitamin D. In adults, a high intake of these fish is associated with better cognitive functions and reduced risk of cardiovascular diseases. According to the Avon Longitudinal Study of Parents and Children, maternal high consumption of fish during pregnancy is associated with less depressive and anxious symptoms in the mother and many positive outcomes in the offspring, including:

- A lower risk of intrauterine growth retardation

- Better communication skills at 15 months of age

- Higher visual-spatial ability at 3 years of age

- Better fine motor skills and social development at 3.5 years of age

- More altruistic behavior at 7 years of age

- A higher verbal IQ at 8 years of age

Other studies have shown that maternal high consumption of fish during pregnancy is associated with lower risk of ADHD in the offspring at 8 years of age.

21. Seafood may be contaminated by mercury, should I still eat it frequently?

Predatory fish such as swordfish, shark, king mackerel, marlin, orange roughy, tuna, and tilefish may be contaminated with heavy, neurotoxic elements like mercury. This is because in aquatic environments, some bacteria can methylate inorganic mercury into methylmercury, which bioaccumulates in marine organisms. It is further biomagnified through the food chain and in humans: the more fish consumption, the higher the blood levels of mercury.

Several studies showed that higher maternal blood levels of mercury during pregnancy was associated with delayed psychomotor development and deficits in attention and verbal skills in the offspring. Nevertheless, surprisingly maternal fish intake during pregnancy was associated with overall positive outcomes in the offspring. Despite being potentially contaminated by mercury, eating fish brings substantial benefits to the infant.

Thus, understandably, seafood high in omega-3 PUFA but low in methylmercury is encouraged and will bring even bigger benefits. Examples of this kind of seafood include salmon, anchovies, herring, shad, sardines, Pacific oysters, trout, Atlantic mackerel, Pacific chub mackerel, shrimp, and scallop (see item 23 for more examples).

22. Can I eat canned seafood?

Better not. A mother-child cohort study in Northeastern Italy by Fabio Barbone at Udine University showed that higher maternal intake of canned fish during pregnancy (servings/week) was associated with a lower nonverbal IQ in the offspring at 7–9 years old. Nonverbal IQ measures nonverbal mental skills, such as the ability to perform picture completion, coding, picture arrangement, block design and object assembly.

The reasons for this negative outcome are severalfold. First, some canned seafood, such as canned white tuna may be particularly high in heavy metals, including methylmercury and lead. Second, some canned seafood, such as anchovies, may be high in sodium. Third, during the industrial processing of canned fish, the nutritional value of the fish is reduced and detrimental changes can occur.

23. How much and what kind of seafood should I eat per week?

The U.S. Department of Health and Human Services recommends that pregnant women should consume 8–12 ounces (227–340 gram, cooked, edible portion) of a variety of seafood per week. This is about 2–3 servings a week. Importantly, seafood choices should be restricted to those lower in methylmercury.

- Preferred choices: anchovy, Atlantic croaker, Atlantic mackerel, black sea bass, butterfish, catfish, clam, cod, crab, crawfish, flounder, haddock, hake, herring, lobster (American and spiny), mullet, Pacific chub mackerel, Pacific oysters, perch (freshwater and ocean), pickerel, plaice, Pollock, salmon, sardines, scallop, skate, shad, shrimp, smelt, sole, squid, tilapia, trout (freshwater), whitefish, whiting

- Try to avoid the following because of the high likelihood of contamination by methylmercury: swordfish, shark, king mackerel, marlin, orange roughy, tuna and tilefish

24. Why should I consume dairy?

Dairy food contains rich nutrients including protein, calcium, monounsaturated fatty acids, vitamin A, the B-group vitamins, vitamin D, iodine, choline, potassium, magnesium, zinc and insulin-like growth factor I. Milk is considered the only food that contains approximately all the essential nutrients that human need.

Research has shown that high intake of dairy food reduces the risk of hypertension, cancer, and diabetes. During pregnancy, maternal high intake of yogurt has been associated with low levels of depressive symptoms.

But since dairy food also contains saturated fatty acids, which are high in calories and raise blood cholesterol levels, it is recommended that choices of dairy food should be fat-free or low-fat (1%).

25. How much and what kind of dairy should I consume every day?

The U.S. Department of Agriculture and Department of Health and Human Services recommend 3 cups of fat-free or low-fat dairy food per day for all adults. Fat-free or low-fat dairy food includes milk, yogurt, milk-based desserts, cheese, and/or fortified soy beverages. Foods such as cream cheese, cream, and butter which are made from milk but have no or little calcium are not counted as dairy foods. 1 cup of dairy food is equivalent to:

- 1 cup (8 fluid ounces or 237 ml) of milk, yogurt, or soymilk (soy beverage)

- 1 cup pudding made with milk

- 1.5 cups ice cream (1 scoop of ice cream is equivalent to 1/3 cup of milk)

- 1.5 ounces (43g) of natural cheese, or 2 ounces (57g) of processed cheese

It must be noted that sweetened dairy products (flavored milk, yogurt, drinkable yogurt, desserts) contain added sugars and may count against your limit for calories.

26. What is the consequence of a "western" diet?

A "western" diet is characterized by high intake of red, processed meat (e.g., sausages, luncheon meats, bacon, and beef jerky, which are products preserved by smoking, curing, salting, and the addition of chemical preservatives), fast foods (high in fat and salt), refined grains, sweets, soft drinks, and salty snacks. That is, it is characterized by high-saturated fats, sugar, and salt.

In the general population, high intake of red, processed meat has been associated with increased risk of cardiovascular diseases, cancer, and diabetes. High intake of fast foods, sweets, soft drinks and salty snacks has been associated with obesity.

During pregnancy, a maternal western diet has been associated with:

- A higher risk of gestational diabetes mellitus

- Higher levels of maternal stress and depressive symptom both during and after pregnancy

- Higher risk of a small for gestational-age infant (indicating restricted fetal growth)

- More externalizing problems (aggressive behaviors, ADHD) at 1.5 and 3 years of age in the offspring

Furthermore, maternal high intake of sweets and soft drinks is associated with excessive weight gain and increased risk of offspring obesity.

27. What is the consequence of a high-fat diet?

A high-fat diet is a diet with its calories provided through a substantial proportion of fat, primarily saturated fat. Typical examples of a high-fat diet include burgers, pizza, and other junk foods. A diet high in fat increases systemic inflammation and is a well-known risk factor for obesity, metabolic syndrome, coronary heart disease and type 2 diabetes. During pregnancy, high maternal inflammation has been linked to many mental health and behavioral disorders in the offspring including depression, anxiety, ADHD, and autism spectrum disorders.

In animals, maternal high-fat diet during pregnancy has been shown to cause placental dysfunction, increase anxiety behavior, prolong stress response, reduce cognitive abilities, and impair social behaviors in the offspring. It also enhances the offspring's preferences for diets with a high-fat content, and increases adiposity. Neurobiologically, this diet alters the gene expression of dopamine (a neurotransmitter involved in working memory, motivation, and reward learning) and opioid-related (involved in reward processing) genes, reduces serotonin (a neurotransmitter involved in stress and emotion regulation) neurotransmission, and changes the receptor expression of the stress hormone cortisol.

28. Is being obese bad for me?

Overweight ($25 \leq$ BMI < 30) and obesity (BMI ≥ 30) increase the levels of cortisol and pro-inflammatory factors, which damage the body and brain. Overweight and obesity have been associated with increased risks of cardiovascular diseases and type 2 diabetes. It has also been estimated that obese people have brain ages that are ten years older than their natural biological age. As a result, overweight and obesity bring many cognitive, emotional and social problems (for more detailed discussion, see Chapter 12 of my recent book *Plato's Insight: How Physical Exercise Boosts Mental Excellence*).

During pregnancy, maternal overweight and obesity cause many complications. In the case of obesity (BMI ≥ 30), it has been associated with:

- An over 3 times higher risk of gestational diabetes mellitus

- A 3–10 times higher risk of pre-eclampsia (a condition characterized by high blood pressure and damage to another organ system such as the liver and kidneys)

- A 4.5–8.7 times higher risk of gestational hypertension

- Induction of labor, prolonged labor and failure to progress

- More than double higher risk of instrumental and cesarean birth

- More than double higher risk of surgical site infection

- Longer stay in hospital

- A 1.4 times higher risk of developing depression and anxiety

29. Is being obese bad for my baby?

Obesity is the result of excessive calories intake. It is also associated with micronutrient deficiencies because of the poor nutritional quality of the food consumed.

Not only that, maternal obesity increases the levels of cortisol, induces a pro-inflammatory status in the body and reduces the levels of BDNF. As a result, maternal obesity during pregnancy is associated with endothelial and placental dysfunction and has been linked to:

- A 1.87 times higher risk of neural tube defect

- A 1.3 times higher risk of fetal death and miscarriage

- A 1.4–2 times higher risk of stillbirth

- An over 1.5 times higher risk of preterm birth

- A 1.2–1.4 times higher risk of low birth weight

- An over 2 times higher risk of large for gestational age infants (indicating risks of obesity)

- A 1.38 times higher risk of neonatal intensive care use

- A lower intention, initiation, and continuation of breastfeeding

- An over 3 times higher risk of childhood overweight/obesity in the offspring

- More attention problems at school at 5 years of age in the offspring

- A 2 times higher risk of emotional problems at school at 5 years of age in the offspring

- A 1.7 times higher risk of ADHD at 7 years of age in the offspring

30. How much gestational weight gain is healthy and why?

The U.S. Institute of Medicine recommends that during pregnancy, women (mothers of singletons) gain different weight according to their basal weight, specifically:

- Underweight women (BMI < 18.5) gain 12.5–18.0 kg

- Healthy weight women (18.5 ≤ BMI < 25) gain 11.5–16 kg

- Overweight women (25 ≤ BMI < 30) gain 7–11.5 kg

- Obese women (BMI ≥ 30) gain 5–9 kg

Typically, women should gain ~1–2 kg during the first trimester, and the rate of weight gain during the second and third trimesters should be steady and different according to their basal weight:

- Underweight women: at a rate of 0.5 kg/week

- Healthy weight women: at a rate of 0.4 kg/week

- Overweight women: at a rate of 0.3 kg/week

- Obese women: at a rate of 0.2 kg/week

Gestational weight gain below or above the recommendation can cause negative outcomes. Gestational weight gain below the recommendation is associated with a 1.70 times higher risk of preterm birth and a 1.53 times higher risk of small for gestational age. Gestational weight gain above the recommendation is associated with a 1.30 times higher risk of cesarean delivery, a 1.85 times higher risk of large for gestational age, and a 1.95 times higher risk of macrosomia (birth weight more than 4,000 grams).

The negative outcomes are particularly high when pre-conceptional obesity is combined with excessive gestational weight gain. In one study, children born to women who were both overweight and gained excessive weight during pregnancy were at a 2.10 times higher risk of ADHD.

For mothers of twins, the U.S. Institute of Medicine recommends:

- Healthy weight women gain 16.8–24.5 kg

- Overweight women gain 14.1–22.7 kg

- Obese women gain 11.3–19.1 kg

For underweight mothers of twins and mothers of multiples, no guideline is available at this stage.

31. How can I deal with obesity and prevent excessive weight gain during pregnancy?

As we have mentioned in item 11, even you are overweight or obese, dieting during pregnancy is not recommended. The primary goal of weight management during pregnancy is to limit weight gain rather than weight loss.

The reason for excessive weight gain is excessive energy intake, especially from high-fat and sugar food, and lack of physical exercise. Thus, the key to preventing obesity and excessive weight gain is to consume appropriate energy, which can be achieved through a lifestyle change, specifically via:

- Eating a healthy, balanced diet: adhere to the Mediterranean-style diet and be familiar with the specific nutritional requirement (e.g., iron, folate, vitamin D) during pregnancy. This can start from displacing energy-dense, nutrient-poor foods with nutritious and wholesome alternatives (see item 33), learning to read food labels and being familiar with the nutritional value of everyday foods, and eating mindfully (see item 34).

- Engaging in physical exercise: attend to safe physical exercise regularly (see item 55).

- Monitoring body weight: be familiar with weight gain targets (see item 30) and monitor your progress.

- Mental health promotion: try to boost positive emotions and create a psychological stress-free environment, as psychological stress and negative emotions destroy a healthy lifestyle and produce toxic chemicals in your body (for more detailed discussion, see *Psychology for Pregnancy*).

Research shows that this kind of lifestyle change improves diet quality, prevents excessive weight gain, and reduces anxiety, the incidence of gestational diabetes mellitus and hypertension and the risk of cesarean delivery and macrosomia, among other things in pregnant women, particularly in those who are obese.

32. What foods help deal with stress and prevent depression?

The answer is seafood especially fatty fish, because fatty fish contains high levels of omega-3 PUFA DHA and EPA. Animal experiments have shown that DHA supplementation reduces animal's stress response including attenuated increases in heart rate, blood pressure, and anxiety in response to stressful events. In humans, it has been reported that, in the face of a difficult academic examination, college students with high blood levels of omega-3 PUFA exhibited reduced increase in pro-inflammatory cytokines.

During pregnancy, high consumption of seafood, especially fatty fish and high blood levels of DHA, are associated with lower levels of maternal depression both during pregnancy and postpartum. Randomized controlled trials (RCTs, a scientifically sound methodology) suggest that supplementation of omega-3 PUFA particularly DHA and EPA in the form of fish oil exerts antidepressant effects in clinically depressed patients.

33. How to successfully start a healthy diet change?

Perhaps one of the easiest and most effective ways to start a healthy diet change is replacing one or two unhealthy food items with healthier food items. You may substitute a food or beverage for another one within the same food group such as:

- Replacing sugar-sweetened beverages with water, fruit juices, yogurt, or milk

- Replacing sweets, potato chips and other high-fat, salty snacks with fruits, healthier snacks or dietary fiber supplements

- Replacing mayonnaise with fresh avocado on a sandwich to reduce saturated fats while adding essential nutrients

- Replacing nutrient-poor salad dressings with an avocado and yogurt-based dressing

- Replacing red, processed meat with salmon (for example, if you eat red meat three times a week, you may try to replace one meal with salmon)

Research has shown this simple substitution approach results in marked improvement in diet quality.

34. What is mindful eating and why is it important?

Today, many people eat mindlessly; some eat while playing smartphone games or watching TV or videos; others eat more sweets and junk food when stressed (which is called emotional eating); still, others eat in response to environmental cues rather than physiological hunger: research shows that the more snacks and soft drinks people keep on their kitchen counters, the more likely they will be obese.

These kinds of mindless eating not only cause overconsumption and lead to obesity, but also cause malnutrition since most of the foods consumed are energy-dense and nutrient-poor. This can be prevented if one eats mindfully rather than mindlessly.

In *Psychology for Pregnancy*, we have introduced the benefits of being mindful, namely intentionally attending to our own experiences with an open and non-judging attitude. Mindful eating involves attending to taste, hunger, and satiety cues and being aware of physical and emotional sensations with a non-judgmental attitude while eating. It is associated with slow pace of eating without distractions (e.g., eating while watching TV), acknowledging bodily sensational responses to food, and increasing awareness of emotional eating. Mindful eating promotes healthy eating such as increasing the consumption of vegetables and decreasing that of fast food, and prevents overconsumption.

During pregnancy, maternal training with mindful eating and yoga (physical postures with meditation and breathing techniques) helps with glycemic control among those with gestational diabetes and reduces the risk of excessive weight gain.

You can take the *Mindful Eating Questionnaire* at https://brainandlife.net/test-mindful-eating to check your levels of eating mindfully and see how you can improve it.

PART 3: NUTRITION SUPPLEMENTATION

35. What supplements should I take during pregnancy and why?

During pregnancy, accompanying the fast development of the fetal body and brain, the nutritional requirement increases substantially and this can only be fulfilled by the mother's intake. However, pure intake through regular diet is not enough, particularly in the case of several micronutrients including folate acid and iron. To assure the optimal development of the fetus, nutrient supplementation should be considered.

Currently WHO recommends:

- Daily supplementation of 30 to 60 mg of iron plus 400 μg folic acid starting from 2 months before the planned pregnancy and throughout pregnancy for all pregnant women to prevent neural tube defects and anemia, and promote maternal and fetal health.

- For those with anemia (blood hemoglobin level lower than 110 g/L), daily supplementation of 120 mg of iron until their blood hemoglobin levels rise to normal (after which they can resume the standard daily 30 to 60 mg of iron).

Supplementation can be fulfilled in the form of fortified foods (foods to which extra nutrients have been added) and/or supplements. This recommendation has been a standard practice around the world.

For other micronutrients, it is generally believed that if pregnant women consume a healthy balanced diet, the intake of micronutrients will be sufficient and there is no need to take further supplements, particularly for those in well-resourced areas such as North America and Europe. In contrast, in low and middle-income countries, where women are more likely to be malnourished, multiple micronutrient supplements including folate acid, iron, and other micronutrients may be preferred (see item 39).

Nevertheless, the objective of WHO is to develop broadly applying guidelines directed towards reducing maternal and neonatal mortality, restricted growth, low birth weight, and preterm birth, and improve maternal satisfaction. WHO has not developed any guideline on how to boost the fetal brain and enhance its intellectual, emotional, and social development after birth, although there have been many studies conducted to investigate this purpose (see item 40 and 41).

36. Introduction to nutrients (1): Folic acid

Folic acid is a B vitamin that plays an important role in DNA synthesis. It is particularly important for the development of the fetal spine, brain, and skull during the first four weeks of pregnancy.

Low folic acid levels around the time of conception may cause neural tube defects in infants. Neural tube defects involve the failure of the neural tube to close properly and typically occur during the third and fourth week of pregnancy, before the woman knows she is pregnant. Research shows that this risk is substantially reduced (by over 70%) when the mother takes daily folic acid supplementation starting from three months before pregnancy continuing up to the 6th week from the beginning of her last menses. Furthermore, the Generation R Study showed that higher maternal blood levels of folate concentration at 13 weeks of gestation were associated with faster fetal head growth, which was independent of overall fetal growth.

WHO recommends a daily supplement containing 400 μg folic acid starting from 2 months before the planned pregnancy and throughout pregnancy for all pregnant women to prevent neural tube defects and anemia and promote maternal and fetal health.

Maternal peri-conception folic acid supplementation has been associated with many positive developmental outcomes in the offspring, including:

- Larger prenatal head size (indicating a bigger and more powerful brain)

- A 65% reduced risk of internalizing problems (e.g., anxiety, depression, withdrawn) and a 45% reduced risk of externalizing problems (e.g., aggression) at 18 months of age

- Higher receptive language ability (namely the ability to understand incoming information) and a 45% reduced risk of severe language delay at 3 years of age

- Higher verbal, motor and executive skills, higher social competence and less attention problems at 4 years of age

- A 39% reduced risk of autism spectrum disorder (characterized by social problems including lack of interest in interacting with others) between 3–10 years of age

37. Introduction to nutrients (2): Iron

Iron, an essential micronutrient, is necessary not only in synthesizing hemoglobin for carrying oxygen but also for forming enzymes that catalyze many processes including the biosynthesis of hormones, synapses, neurotransmission, and DNA and RNA base repair.

Iron requirements during pregnancy increase substantially due to increased requirements by the placenta and the fetus. Unfortunately, about 42% of pregnant women around the world, that is, almost one in two pregnant women are anemic. Even in well-resourced areas such as North America and Europe, the prevalence of anemia is as high as 25%, or one in four pregnant women. Half of the anemia is due to iron deficiency.

Iron deficiency during pregnancy has been associated with:

- Poor auditory recognition memory as evaluated by the ability to differentiate the mother's voices from a stranger's voices at birth

- High levels of negative emotionality (distress) and low levels of alertness and soothability after birth

- Low psychomotor development at 1 year of age

- Deficits in the ability to recall multi-step event sequences at 1–4 years of age

- Poor language ability, low fine motor skills, and impaired attention at 5 years of age

WHO recommends daily supplements of 30 to 60 mg of iron plus 400 μg folic acid starting from 2 months before pregnancy and throughout pregnancy for all pregnant women, whereas for those with anemia the recommendation is daily 120 mg of iron until their blood hemoglobin levels rise to normal (after which they can resume the standard daily 30 to 60 mg of iron).

A recent study by Parul Christian at Johns Hopkins University reported that maternal supplementation with iron and folic acid at the amount recommended by WHO during pregnancy:

- Increased nonverbal IQ (involving problem-solving abilities using visual information and motor skills) by 2.38 points in the offspring at 7–9 years of age

Even after finishing the above recommended supplementation, pregnant women are encouraged to eat iron-rich foods throughout pregnancy and after delivery.

- Iron-rich animal foods include lean red meat such as beef and lamb, and seafood such as sardines, perch, and oysters

- Iron-rich plant foods include dark green leafy vegetables (e.g., spinach and broccoli), legumes (e.g., beans, soybeans, and peas), tofu, and iron-fortified cereals, breads and pastas

Note that iron is 4–6 times better absorbed from animal foods than plant foods and that eating vitamin C-containing foods such as vegetables, fruit and fruit juices with meals increases iron absorption from plant foods.

38. Introduction to nutrients (3): Vitamin D

Vitamin D plays an important role in bone metabolism through regulation of calcium and phosphate homeostasis. It also has immune-modulating effects and is a regulator of gene expression.

Vitamin D is mainly produced by the body during exposure to sunlight (skin synthesis), but is also found in oily fish (e.g., salmon, herring, perch, and trout, etc.), eggs, liver, some mushrooms, and fortified dairy products (e.g., milk in which extra vitamin D is added).

The main risk factors of vitamin D deficiency are insufficient sunlight exposure and inadequate diet. Dark pigmentation, dark skin color, clothing that limits the exposure of skin to sunlight, long hours working indoors, avoidance of sunshine for reducing the risk of skin cancer, winter seasons, and environmental pollution all inhibit the synthesis of vitamin D in the skin. Vitamin D deficiency during pregnancy has been linked to:

- A 5 times higher risk of pre-eclampsia

- A 2.66 times higher risk of gestational diabetes mellitus

- Higher risk of preterm birth

- A 2.4 times higher risk of small for gestational age infants

Vitamin D supplementation during pregnancy improves maternal vitamin D status and reduces the risk of the above conditions. However, in the most recent guideline, WHO recommends pregnant women receive an adequate intake of vitamin D primarily through the consumption of a healthy balanced diet. For those at risk, for example, with little sunlight exposure, living at northern latitude, dark-skin, vegan-vegetarian diet, vitamin D screening is recommended.

Vitamin D status is most commonly assessed through the measurement of circulating vitamin D, known as serum 25-hydroxyvitamin D (25(OH) D or calcidiol) levels. The U.S. Institute of Medicine defines levels of serum 25(OH)D greater than 50 nmol/L (or 20 ng/mL) as adequate for pregnant women. Pregnant women with levels of serum 25(OH)D below this should consult with doctors or other healthcare professionals to take vitamin D supplementation.

39. Introduction to nutrients (4): Multiple micronutrient supplements

Due to inadequate diet, many pregnant women in low and middle-income countries suffer from multiple nutrient deficiencies as dietary intake alone cannot meet micronutrient requirements in pregnancy. In 1999, the United Nations Children's Fund (UNICEF), WHO, and United Nations University proposed the United Nations International Multiple Micronutrient Preparation (UNIMMAP) containing 15 micronutrients for pregnant women in low and middle-income countries. This daily multiple micronutrient supplements (MMS) consist of:

- Iron 30 mg

- Folic acid 400 µg

- Zinc 15 mg

- Copper 2.0 mg

- Selenium 65 µg

- Vitamin A 800 µg retinol equivalent

- Vitamin B1 1.4 mg

- Vitamin B2 1.4 mg

- Niacin 18 mg

- Vitamin B6 1.9 mg

- Vitamin B12 2.6 µg

- Vitamin C 70 mg

- Vitamin D 5 µg

- Vitamin E 10 mg

- Iodine 150 µg

All these micronutrients are essential for healthy fetal development. For instance, vitamin A, whose active form is called retinol, is best known for its role in color and night vision and is also involved in immune function (anti-inflammatory), bone metabolism and blood production. It is a fat-soluble vitamin rich in liver, kidney, eggs, and dairy foods. It has been reported that maternal supplementation of vitamin A during pregnancy reduces the risk of maternal night blindness, clinical infection, and anemia, while maternal antenatal and newborn supplementation combined together boost the offspring's performance in reading, spelling and math at 8 years of age.

Iodine is required for the synthesis of thyroid hormones, which are required for regulating cell metabolism. The primary dietary sources of iodine are dairy foods, bread, seafood, meat and iodised salt. A meta-analysis of 37 studies involving over 12,000 children born and raised in China before and after national iodine food fortification found that children exposed to severe iodine deficiency lost 12.45 IQ points, with 8.7 IQ points recovered with iodine supplementation.

MMS was intended for replacing the standard iron-folate supplements, although up until now research is still ongoing to confirm the superiority of MMS. A 2017 meta-analysis of 17 trials involving 137,791 women reported that compared to the standard iron-folate supplements, MMS reduces the risk of low birth weight by 12% and small for gestational age by 8%.

Meanwhile, the Supplementation with Multiple Micronutrients Intervention Trial (SUMMIT), a double-blind cluster-randomized trial conducted in Indonesia led by public health specialist Anuraj H. Shankar at Harvard University, found more benefits with MMS. MMS, which was provided throughout pregnancy until three months postpartum:

- Improved maternal cognitive ability (The effect size was equivalent to one year of education for all mothers; in anemic mothers, the effect size was equivalent to two years of education; in undernourished mothers as defined by mid upper arm circumference less than 23.5 cm, the effect size was equivalent to three years of education)

- Improved maternal reading efficiency (This is important as we will see in Volume 3 of this series that parental early reading to their child promotes the development of language abilities and academic achievement of the child)

- Reduced early infant mortality by 18%

- Reduced the risk of low birth weight by 14%

- Boosted procedural memory in offspring between 9–12 years of age (Procedural memory underlies the learning of perceptual, motor, and cognitive skills; the effect size was equivalent to half a year of school education)

- Improved IQ in the offspring born to anemic mothers between 9–12 years of age (The effect size was equivalent to that by one year of school education)

40. Introduction to nutrients (5): Omega-3 PUFA

Approximately 50–60% of the dry adult brain weight is fatty acids, of which a large proportion is the omega-3 PUFA including α-linolenic acid (ALA), DHA and EPA. They are essential for the production of neurons and synapses, and have anti-inflammatory properties.

Contrary to saturated and monounsaturated fatty acids, omega-3 PUFA cannot be synthesized in the human body and are therefore considered essential nutrients. (Although within omega-3 PUFA, ALA can be converted to DHA and EPA, the conversion rate is very low in humans.)

During pregnancy, PUFAs are transferred from the mother to the fetus and maternal intake of PUFA determines how much is available to the fetus for brain growth. The availability of PUFA to the fetus during pregnancy is critical for optimal neurocognitive development. For instance, maternal blood levels of DHA during pregnancy or at birth have been associated with offspring:

- Better attentional functioning at 2 years of age

- Less emotional problems between 5–6 years of age

- Higher full-scale IQ at 6.5 and 8 years of age

Furthermore, maternal daily supplementation of DHA alone or together with EPA during pregnancy (from the second trimester to birth or 3 months after birth) has been associated with:

- High levels of sustained attention across the first year

- Better language development (more words understood and produced) at 14 and 18 months of age

- Higher ability for eye and hand coordination at 2.5 years of age

- Over 4 points higher in IQ at 4 years of age

The European Commission charged the European research projects Perinatal Lipid Metabolism and Early Nutrition Programming to develop recommendations on dietary fat intake during pregnancy and lactation. After an extensive review of the scientific evidence, these projects established that:

- Pregnant and lactating women require at least 200 mg of DHA per day.

- Dietary intakes up to 1 gram DHA per day or 2.7 gram EPA plus DHA per day have been used in clinical trials without significant adverse effects.

However, the average daily intake of DHA throughout westernized countries is much lower than that is required and estimated to be about 150 mg per day. Thus, pregnant women should try to increase the intake of DHA and EPA, through consumption of seafood (particularly fatty fish such as salmon, herring, trout) or fish oil supplements.

41. Introduction to nutrients (6): The ratio of omega-6 to omega-3 PUFA

PUFA has two families, omega-3 and omega-6. Omega-6 PUFA includes linoleic acid and arachidonic acid (AA). Dietary sources of omega-6 PUFA include plant oils such as sunflower, safflower, corn oils, soybean oils, nuts, and seeds.

High consumption of omega-6 PUFA has been associated with low inflammation and low risk of cardiovascular diseases, type 2 diabetes, and cancer. During pregnancy, maternal low blood levels of AA have been associated with low nonverbal IQ of the offspring at 8 years of age.

However, omega-6 PUFA competes for the same desaturase enzymes in the biosynthetic pathways to omega-3 PUFA. Therefore, high intake of omega-6 PUFA results in a low omega-3 PUFA status. This is further emphasized in people with low intake of omega-3 PUFA, that is, low intake of fatty fish or without fish oil supplements.

In animal experiments, a high maternal omega-6: omega-3 ratio diet during pregnancy has been found to impair neurogenesis (production of neurons) after birth and increase anxiety-like behavior in adulthood in the offspring.

Meanwhile, in humans, a lower maternal omega-6: omega-3 ratio in the blood or diet (that is, a higher omge-3: omega-6 diet) during pregnancy has been associated with offspring:

- Faster cognitive development at 6 months of age

- Faster psychomotor development at 6 and 9 months of age

- Greater language ability at 2 years of age

- Better overall development (including communication, motor, problem-solving, and social) at 3 years of age

- Fewer emotional problems (depression, anxiety) and lower risk of ADHD at 5–6 years of age

- Fewer symptoms of autism at 6 years of age

Whereas the ratio of omega-6: omega-3 in today's diet is estimated to be 10–20:1, a target of 1–2:1 is preferred. Therefore, it is recommended that when increasing the intake of omega-6 PUFA, you also increase the consumption of seafood rich in omega-3 PUFA or take fish oil supplements.

PART 4: FOOD SAFETY & SUBSTANCE ABUSE

42. Can I drink coffee and tea during pregnancy?

Yes, you can, but as little as possible. The American College of Obstetricians and Gynecologists recommends that pregnant women or women trying to become pregnant should consume no more than 200 mg of caffeine per day. This amount is about one 12-oz (350 ml) cup of coffee.

Coffee, tea, energy drinks, and some soft drinks contain caffeine. At moderate doses, caffeine exerts stimulatory effects by blocking adenosine receptors in the brain particular in the cerebral cortex, hippocampus, and cerebellum. However, over-stimulation of neurons is toxic and may cause neuronal death.

During pregnancy, caffeine metabolism is slowed down in the mother and caffeine crosses placenta and reaches the fetus, which raises the concern about its potential risks on the fetal brain. Meanwhile, coffee and coffee products contain the carcinogen and neurotoxic agent acrylamide, which further emphasizes the risk (see item 43).

Animal experiments have shown that:

- A very high dose of maternal daily caffeine intake during pregnancy is associated with reduced offspring cerebral weight;

- Maternal caffeine intake equivalent to 6–9 cups of coffee per day in humans causes depression-like behavior in the offspring at adulthood;

- Maternal caffeine intake equivalent to 2–3 cups of coffee per day in humans impairs object recognition memory and working memory in the offspring at adulthood.

In humans, regular caffeine intake during pregnancy has been associated with:

- Increased risk of neural tube defects

- *At birth*: poorer neuromuscular development and reflex functioning, heightened arousal and irritability

- *At 18 months of age*: hyperactivity

- *At 4-9 years of age*: over 4 times higher risk of social problems

43. Why should I stop eating fried potato chips and cookies?

Fried potato chips are typical salty snacks low in nutrients and high in calories and fat. Worse than that, fried potato chips contain the highest concentrations of acrylamide. Acrylamide is a chemical created when cooked at high temperatures and is a proven carcinogen and neurotoxic agent. Dietary intake of acrylamide increases the risk of breast and kidney cancer. Tobacco smoke and the following foods are high in acrylamide:

- Potato products: potato chips, French fries, and potato snacks

- Cereals: breakfast cereals, roasted cereals

- Baked goods: crisp bread, salty sticks, cookies, biscuits

- Coffee and coffee products

In humans, intake of potato chips increases inflammation in the body. In animals, feeding fried potato chips to female rats during pregnancy induces neuronal death in the offspring brain and causes delayed growth.

44. How can soft cheese, raw sprouts, and melons be dangerous?

Soft cheese made with unpasteurized milk and raw sprouts may contain high levels of the bacterium Listeria monocytogenes, which causes Listeria infection or Listeriosis.

It has been estimated that pregnant women are 10 times more likely than other people to develop Listeria infection while pregnant Hispanic women are 24 times more likely to develop Listeria infection.

Listeria infection may only cause mild illness in the mother including fever, flu-like (fatigue and muscle aches) or gastrointestinal symptoms (diarrhea), but it is devastating to the fetus. Only a single bacterium is required to cause placental infection. Listeria infection during pregnancy may cause miscarriage, stillbirth, preterm birth, spontaneous abortion, neonatal infection, and neonatal death.

To reduce the risk of Listeria infection, you should avoid or be very careful of the consumption of high risk foods:

- *Unpasteurized dairy products including soft cheeses*: Avoid eating soft cheese unless it is labeled as made with pasteurized milk. Soft cheeses made with unpasteurized milk are estimated to be 50 to 160 times more likely to cause Listeria infection than those made with pasteurized milk.

- *Raw sprouts*: Sprouts need warm and humid conditions to sprout and grow and unfortunately, these conditions are also ideal for the growth of bacteria, including Listeria, Salmonella, and E. coli. Do not eat raw or lightly cooked sprouts of any kind (including alfalfa, clover, radish, and mung bean sprouts). Cook sprouts thoroughly to kill the harmful bacteria. When you eat a ready-made sandwich, salad, or Asian foods, make sure it doesn't contain any raw sprouts. Note that rinsing sprouts will not remove bacteria.

- *Melons*: Eat cut melon right away or refrigerate it at 5 °C or colder and for no more than 7 days; do not eat cut melons left at room temperature for more than 4 hours.

- *Hot dogs, pâtés, lunch meats, and cold cuts*: Avoid eating hot dogs, lunch meats, cold cuts, other deli meats (such as bologna), or fermented or dry sausages unless they are heated to an internal temperature of 74 °C or until steaming hot just before serving. Do not eat refrigerated pâté or meat spreads from a deli or meat counter or from the refrigerated section of a store; refrigerate canned or shelf-stable pâté and meat spreads after opening.

- *Avoid cross-contaminating*: Don't let fluid/juice from hot dog and lunch meat packages get on other foods, utensils, and food preparation surfaces. Wash all utensils and surfaces after preparing meat dishes or cutting prepared foods. Wash hands after handling hot dogs, lunch meats, and deli meats.

- *Smoked seafood*: Do not eat refrigerated smoked seafood unless it is canned (although you should also limit the intake of canned seafood, see item 22) or shelf-stable (it can be safely stored at room temperature or "on the shelf") or it is in a cooked dish, such as a casserole.

45. How dangerous is smoking for me?

Very dangerous.

There are over 4,000 chemicals in cigarette smoke including benzo(a)pyrene, nicotine, carbon monoxide and acrylamide, and many are carcinogens. Cigarette smoking, whether active or passive (second-hand smoking), substantially increases the risk of various cancers (such as lung cancer, oral cancer, laryngeal cancer, esophageal cancer, stomach cancer, cancer of the urinary bladder, pancreatic cancer, kidney cancer, cervical cancer, breast cancer, colorectal cancer, and liver cancer), cardiovascular diseases (coronary heart disease), respiratory diseases (COPD), dental diseases, cataract and macular degeneration, peptic ulcer disease, fractures, osteoporosis, and diabetes.

During pregnancy, smoking causes many complications, including but not limited to:

- A 1.67 times higher risk of preterm rupture of membrane

- A 1.65 times higher risk of chorioamnionitis

- A 1.63 times higher risk of incompetent cervix

- A 1.38 times higher risk of threatened premature delivery

- A 1.37 times higher risk of placental abruption

- A 1.20 times higher risk of pregnancy-induced hypertension

- A 1.23 times higher risk of stillbirth

46. Does smoking affect my baby?

Many of the toxic chemicals cross the placenta and due to poor metabolism of the fetus, many chemicals turn out to be higher in concentration in the fetus than in the maternal body. For instance, it has been estimated that the fetal concentration of nicotine is 15% higher than that in the maternal body. These toxic chemicals have direct detrimental effects on the fetal brain and body. Furthermore, nicotine increases maternal blood pressure and heart rate and induces vasoconstriction of the uteroplacental vasculature, which reduces fetal blood circulation and in turn decreases the nutrients and oxygen available to the fetus. Finally, nicotine suppresses maternal appetite, which causes poor nutrition of the mother and fetus.

Maternal smoking during pregnancy has been linked to a higher risk of fetal defects, including:

- A 1.98 times higher risk of atrial septal defects

- A 1.27 times higher risk of gastrointestinal defects

- A 1.25 times higher risk of eye defects

Offspring of mothers who smoked during pregnancy has:

- *At fetal period*: a smaller volume of the cerebellum and ventricular system

- *At birth*: a smaller volume of the cerebellum and frontal lobe

- *At 10–13 years*: a reduced gray matter (consisting of neuronal cell bodies) volume of the cerebral cortex

As a result, children whose mothers smoked during pregnancy have poorer cognitive development:

- The Danish National Birth Cohort found that at 5 years of age, children of mothers who smoked >=10 cigarettes per day during pregnancy had 4 lower IQ points than those of non-smoking mothers;

- The Swedish Cohort Study found that at 15 years of age, adolescents of mothers who smoked 1–9 cigarettes per day during pregnancy were 1.6 times more likely to perform poorly at school, whereas those of mothers who smoked >=10 cigarettes per day were 1.9 times more likely to perform poorly. (These findings do not suggest 9 cigarettes per day are equally toxic as 1 cigarette per day and that 20 cigarettes per day are equally toxic as 10 cigarettes per day. We know that the more cigarettes smoked, the more dangerous.)

Thus, cigarettes should be avoided all together.

This reduced cognitive development and poor academic achievement in the offspring of mothers who smoked during pregnancy have been confirmed in several large scale studies conducted in the United States, Canada, Australia, Spain, Taiwan, Poland, and South Korea. These studies further found that:

- The offspring of mothers who smoked during pregnancy exhibit various emotional and social problems: they are more impulsive, aggressive, more likely to experience negative emotions such as depression, at a higher risk of ADHD, and have more problems with peers;

- The offspring of mothers who smoked during pregnancy are at a 1.35 times higher risk of overweight, and a 1.28 times higher risk of obesity;

- Smoking by the father or other household members at home when the mother does not smoke has similar detrimental effects on the development of the offspring.

47. Should family members stop smoking during pregnancy?

Absolutely.

As shown by many studies, smoking by the father or other household members at home even when the pregnant mother does not smoke has similar detrimental effects on the development of the offspring. For instance, as estimated by a 2014 meta-analysis, maternal smoking during pregnancy is associated with a 1.35 times higher risk of overweight and a 1.28 times higher risk of obesity in the offspring; in contrast, household smoking by a family member is associated with a 1.22 times higher risk of overweight and a 1.31 times higher risk of obesity in the offspring. In another 2012 study, maternal and paternal smoking during pregnancy had a similar association with offspring ADHD symptoms.

48. Why should I avoid any alcohol?

Fetal alcohol spectrum disorders are a leading cause of developmental disabilities due to maternal alcohol drinking during pregnancy. Affected infants not only show abnormal physical appearance but also exhibit severely delayed cognitive and behavioral development.

It is because that alcohol induces abnormalities in glial cells, the latter provide nutrients to neurons. As a result, alcohol reduces neuronal survival and causes severe damage to the brain.

In an English study of over 9,000 children, Kapil Sayal at the University of Bristol, U.K. found that maternal consumption of even one small drink per week during the first trimester causes clinically significant mental health problems in the offspring at 4 and 7 years of age.

49. Toxic chemicals (1): Cocaine

Cocaine is a drug which blocks the function of monoamine re-uptakes transporters, the latter are not only important for normal neurotransmission but also play pivotal trophic roles in the production of neurons and synapses. Therefore, maternal cocaine use during pregnancy severely impairs the neural development of the fetus. Offspring born to mothers exposed to cocaine during pregnancy:

- *At 4.5 years of age*: more likely to express frustration and show disruptive behavior.

- *At 6 years of age*: more likely to have symptoms of oppositional defiant disorder and ADHD.

- *At 13–15 years of age*: have thinner dorsolateral prefrontal cortex, which is a brain area critical for executive function (i.e., fluid intelligence), and smaller caudate, which is a brain area critical for motivation and reward processing.

- *At 14–17 years of age*: have lower gray matter volume in cortical and limbic regions important for cognitive and emotional processing.

50. Toxic chemicals (2): Cannabis

Cannabis is a drug also called grass, hashish, hemp, marijuana, and pot. It interacts with the endogenous cannabinoid system in the brain and has been shown to exhibit many of the combined effects of alcohol, hallucinogens, opiates, and tranquillizers. Maternal exposure to cannabis has been linked to:

- *At birth*: a 1.77 times higher risk of low birth weight; smaller head circumference (indicating a smaller brain); and a 2.02 times higher risk of placement of the infant in neonatal intensive care unit;

- *At 6 years of age*: deficit in sustained attention;

- *At 10 years of age*: hyperactivity, impulsivity, inattention, increased delinquency and externalizing problems.

51. Toxic chemicals (3): Methamphetamine

In the mother, methamphetamine increases the risk of hypertension, decreases appetite and leads to extreme weight loss. Furthermore, methamphetamine causes vasoconstriction and a restriction of nutrients and oxygen to the fetus. In addition, methamphetamine can across the placenta and cause direct damage to fetal organs.

As a result, the offspring of mothers exposed to methamphetamine during pregnancy have:

- *At birth*: smaller head circumferences; more likely to require neonatal intensive care unit admission; poorer suck ability; exaggerated stress response.

- *At 1 year of age*: poorer grasping ability.

- *At 3 years of age*: poorer grasping ability; increased depression and anxiety.

- *At 4 years of age*: lower IQ.

- *At 5 years of age*: lower executive function (i.e., fluid intelligence); increased depression and anxiety; more impulsive behaviors and aggression; increased ADHD symptoms.

- *At 8 years of age*: more aggressive behaviors and poorer peer relationships.

- *At 14 years of age*: poorer school performance in math and language; more difficulty with physical fitness activities.

Many of these motor, cognitive, and emotional deficits may be explained by reduced brain volumes, such as:

- Smaller putamen (a brain area involved in attention and motor function)

- Smaller globus pallidus (involved in attention and motor function)

- Smaller hippocampus (critical for memory formation and emotion regulation)

PART 5: WORK, PHYSICAL EXERCISE, & ENVIRONMENTAL RISKS

52. Does my job affect my baby?

Yes, most likely. Physical demanding work and long-duration standing limit blood flow, therefore, the supply of oxygen and nutrients to the fetus which may cause poor fetal growth. Also, as we have shown in *Psychology for Pregnancy*, high levels of work-related psychological stress exert negative effects on the fetus. In addition, exposure to occupational noise (see item 53) and chemicals interferes with fetal growth, the size of which varies according to the toxicity of the exposure.

A 2006 meta-analysis by Keith T Palmer at the Medical Research Council, U.K. estimated that:

- Compared to those who work less than 40 hours per week, pregnant women who work for at least 40 hours per week during pregnancy have a 1.31 times higher risk of preterm birth. (This is mostly based on studies on the first two trimesters of pregnancy, since pregnant women generally stop working as pregnancy progresses)

Furthermore, a 2014 meta-analysis by MDM van Beukering at the Department of Occupational Health and Safety Service, The Netherlands estimated that:

- Standing and walking at work for more than 3 hours per day is associated with a 1.41 times higher risk of preterm birth (Note that most studies involved standing and walking for more than 5 hours per day).

- Lifting and carrying > 5 kg during pregnancy (mostly the first trimester) is associated with a 1.24 times higher risk of preterm birth. Specifically, lifting and carrying > 5 kg during the third trimester is associated with a 1.30 times higher risk of preterm birth.

- Jobs require physical effort or physical exertion confer a 1.40 times higher risk of preterm birth.

53. Why should I live and work in a quiet, non-noisy place?

Noise, whether due to road, rail, or air traffic, industries, construction, public work, or just the neighborhood is a typical physical stressor. It induces many negative health effects, including hearing impairment, hypertension, cardiovascular disease, headache, fatigue, irritability, sleep disturbance, dementia, and impaired work performance. In school age children, chronic environmental noise reduces cognitive performance and reading comprehension.

During pregnancy, aircraft noise has been linked to premature birth, whereas occupational noise exposure has been associated with:

- An up to 3 times higher risk of spontaneous abortion

- A 2 times higher risk of preterm birth

- An up to 3.9 times higher risk of low birthweight

- A 1.9 times higher risk of intrauterine growth retardation

In a 2014 animal experiment, compared to those born to mothers raised in a normal, quiet environment, rat pups whose mothers were exposed to 95 dB of sound an hour a day during pregnancy had 30% decreased neurogenesis (production of neurons) in the motor cortex and 11.5% decreased neurogenesis in the somatosensory cortex. Interestingly, rat pups whose mothers were exposed to 65 dB of comfortable music during pregnancy had 30% increased neurogenesis in the motor cortex and 40% increased neurogenesis in the somatosensory cortex.

As we have suggested in *Psychology for Pregnancy*, it is good you listen to slow, soothing music during pregnancy because it not only comforts you and reduces your stress, but also stimulates your baby's developing brain (see Volume 3 of this series).

54. Should I stop shiftwork during pregnancy?

Yes, you should.

Shiftwork or rotating shift work, including night work, disrupts biological circadian rhythms and sleep/wake cycle. As a chronic stressor, shiftwork increases the levels of cortisol and pro-inflammatory cytokines. In the general population, shiftwork is associated with increased risk of many physical and psychological conditions including cardiovascular diseases, cancers, gastrointestinal disorders, type 2 diabetes, depression, and anxiety.

During pregnancy, maternal shiftwork has been associated with:

- A higher risk of pre-eclampsia

- A higher risk of miscarriage

- A 1.24 times higher risk of preterm birth

- A 1.27 times higher risk of low birth weight (as I write this paragraph, an acquaintance who is a nurse and continued shiftwork till the early third trimester of her pregnancy, has just experienced a rupture of membranes and underwent induced labor at 34 weeks' gestation. Her baby was also unfortunately around merely 2100 grams at birth: a low birth weight)

In addition, in animal experiments, maternal circadian disruption during pregnancy has been associated with abnormal offspring development, including:

- Increased anxiety

- Hyperactivity and risk-taking behavior

- Reduced vocalizations

- Impaired spatial learning ability

- Reduced adult hippocampal neurogenesis and synaptic plasticity

- Social avoidance

55. Is physical exercise recommended during pregnancy?

Yes. As long as you are free of health complications, you should exercise regularly.

Regular exercise increases the level of BDNF (which supports the production, growth, differentiation, and survival of neurons) and reduces systemic inflammation. Regular mild to moderate intensity physical exercise not only reduces maternal stress and depression, but also prevents gestational excessive weight gain and many complications. Furthermore, infants born to mothers who engaged in physical exercise for 2.5 hours per week (equivalent to 30 minutes for five days a week) during pregnancy have been found to:

- Be 1.2 times more likely to show high vocabulary ability at 15 months of age.

- Possess higher language ability at 2 years of age.

For more details and guidelines on physical exercise during pregnancy, please refer to *Psychology for Pregnancy* and https://brainandlife.net/exercise.

Here I want to make one revision of what we have discussed in item 2, The seed of intelligence dissected.

We say four pillars are at the core of the nourishing components of an enriched environment and the third pillar is a reduced maternal level of the stress hormone cortisol. Exposure to continuously increasing levels of cortisol damages the brain and causes many physical and psychological problems. This phenomenon is true, but there is an exception: physical exercise. Physical exercise, despite increasing cortisol, benefits almost every aspect of neurocognitive functioning. I termed this phenomenon the *"Exercise-Glucocorticoid Paradox"*, which was the theme of my Ph.D. dissertation. If you are interested and want to read more, please visit https://brainandlife.net and check my research profiles.

56. What are the benefits of utilizing green environments?

Green environments or green spaces include public green areas such as parks, gardens, playgrounds, zoos, open space between buildings such as street trees, and suburban natural areas and forests. They may also include "blue spaces" with water elements ranging from ponds to coastal zones.

Green environments improve air quality (by reducing particle matter and air pollution), buffer noise, increase people's physical activities and social contact, and enhance immune functioning.

Many studies have found that greater exposure to green space, such as living in urban areas with more green space and more time spent in green space (regularly using parks), is associated with higher levels of vitality, lower levels of stress, depression, and anxiety, higher cognitive functioning, faster recovery from psychological stress and physical illness, and reduced risk of cardiovascular morbidity and type 2 diabetes. In one British study, moving to greener areas was associated with mental health improvements persisting to three years following the move. In another American study, having natural elements or settings such as a park, trees, farmland, and animals in view from a window contributed substantially to residents' satisfaction with their neighborhood and mental health.

As related to pregnancy, access to green space in close proximity to one's homes has been reported to reduce the risk of low birth weight and preterm birth.

57. Does air pollution affect me?

Yes. Air pollution consists of a diverse mixture of environmental toxins including particulate matter (PM), gases (e.g. ozone, nitrogen oxides and benzene), organic compounds (e.g. polycyclic aromatic hydrocarbons and endotoxins) and metals (e.g. vanadium and nickel).

Air pollution induces chronic inflammation in the body: it increases the blood levels of pro-inflammatory cytokines. Thus, air pollution has been linked to obesity, and pulmonary and cardiovascular diseases. The increased cytokines also reach the brain and increase the risk of many nervous diseases such as ischemic stroke, Alzheimer disease, and Parkinson's disease.

58. Does air pollution affect my baby?

Yes. The size of the effect depends on the severity of air pollution. Air pollution may cause chronic inflammation in your placenta, which affects the normal growth of your unborn baby. It has been estimated that:

- Per 10 $\mu g/m^3$ increment in maternal exposure to PM2.5 during pregnancy is associated with a 1.09 times increased risk of low birth weight; (The detrimental effect of PM2.5 in areas with severe air pollution is substantial: according to the data of WHO, as in 2015, the highest PM2.5 was 217 $\mu g/m^3$ in Zabol of Iran, which was over 210 ug/ m^3 more than that in Sinclair, Carbon, Wyoming of the U.S., the latter had the lowest PM2.5 of 1.6 $\mu g/m^3$).

- Per 10 ppb increase in maternal ozone exposure is associated with a 1.07 times increased risk of low birth weight and small for gestational age.

- A 10-fold increase in maternal exposure to hexachlorobenzene is associated with an 8.14 times higher risk of obesity and a 4.44 mmHg higher systolic blood pressure at 4 years of age.

- Maternal exposure to high levels of nitrogen dioxide and benzene is associated with reduced infant mental development (Notably, this negative effect is attenuated in those born to mothers with high intake of fruits and vegetables).

- Maternal exposure to high levels of polycyclic aromatic hydrocarbon has been linked to a 2.26 times higher risk of offspring obesity at 7 years of age.

This may be a big problem for people living in areas with severe air pollution. As estimated by WHO, from 2008 to 2013, the global urban air pollution levels increased by 8%. In general, air pollution levels are highest in low and middle-income countries in WHO's Eastern Mediterranean and South-East Asia Regions, which often exceed 5–10 times of the WHO limits.

59. Toxic chemicals (4): Lead

Lead binds strongly to sulfhydryl groups on proteins. In the brain, it interferes with the normal functioning of enzymes and severely impairs energy metabolism, neurotransmission, and brain development. Research has shown that:

Even a very low level of maternal blood lead is associated with delayed mental development in the offspring at 2–3 years of age.

Sources of lead exposure include older housing stock, petrol, paint, artificial turf playing fields, jewelry, some folk (traditional) medicine, lead-contaminated (tap) water, dust, food, and drink.

There is no safe blood lead level that has been identified. Therefore, you should avoid any exposure to lead and any lead hazards in your environment must be identified and removed. You can:

- Regularly wash hands to reduce exposure to contaminated dust or soil

- Clean dusty surfaces of floors, furniture, windowsills etc. regularly with a wet mop to remove contaminated dust

- Remove shoes before entering your house to prevent bringing in lead-contaminated soil

- Avoid playing on bare soil

- Avoid using folk medicine and cosmetics that may contain lead

- Avoid using containers or cookware to cook or store foods that are not shown to be lead-free

- Avoid using jewelry that may contain high levels of lead, such as dull-looking metal, fake pearls with pearlescent coating, plastic or vinyl cords or bracelets, lobster-claw clasps

- Consume iron-rich foods such as lean red meat and dark green leafy vegetables, and take iron supplements. In the gastrointestinal tract, iron and lead compete for the same divalent metal transporter 1 and iron deficiency increases lead uptake

According to the U.S. Center for Disease Control and Prevention, if your house was built before 1978, the paint may have lead unless tests show otherwise. You had better talk to your local health department about testing lead in your house. You should not be present in housing built before 1978 that is undergoing renovation.

To know whether or not you have been poisoned by lead, you can take a blood test.

PART 6: SLEEP

60. What are the typical sleep problems during pregnancy?

During pregnancy, women generally experience increasing sleep problems and report poor sleep quality.

During the first trimester, due to hormone changes, nausea, vomiting, and frequent urination, more light sleep and nighttime awakenings occur. Despite increased total sleep time, daytime sleepiness increases.

During the second trimester, because of the increasing uterine size, the bladder is compressed more severely, which causes more frequent urination. Heartburn and increasing fetal movements further worsen sleep: they cause more nighttime awakenings and fragmented sleep.

During the third trimester, physical changes associated with pregnancy including back pain, hip/pelvic pain, itching, leg cramps, and contractions, as well as psychological worry about labor and delivery impair the pregnant women's ability to fall asleep and maintain sleep. As a result, total sleep time is reduced.

61. How much sleep is necessary?

Although there is individual difference, generally, adults need 7–9 hour of sleep per day. However, several studies suggest that during pregnancy, maternal sleep duration less than 8 hours per night is associated with poor birth outcomes (see item 63). Therefore, 8–9 hours of sleep during pregnancy is preferable.

It must be noted that oversleep (sleep duration > 9 hours) is also detrimental to health, as it increases the risk of obesity.

62. How does insufficient and poor sleep affect me?

Chronic sleep deprivation and poor sleep are chronic stressors. They increase the levels of stress hormone cortisol and pro-inflammatory cytokines and decrease the levels of BDNF. As a result, it impairs your cognitive abilities and causes emotional problems, such as depression and anxiety (for more detailed descriptions, see Chapter 9 of *Plato's Insight: How Physical Exercise Boosts Mental Excellence*).

Several studies have shown that pregnant women who report more insomnia symptoms (such as difficulty in initiating and maintaining sleep, early morning awakening) and/or poor sleep quality (do not feel refreshed after sleep) are more likely to have increased depressive symptoms during pregnancy and develop postpartum depression. Besides, short sleep duration (< 7 hours per night) and/or poor sleep impair carbohydrate metabolism and increase the risk of gestational diabetes mellitus. Finally, short sleep duration (< 7 hours per night) is associated with longer labor duration and high rates of cesarean births.

63. Does my sleep affect my baby?

As insufficient sleep and poor sleep increase the level of stress hormone cortisol and pro-inflammatory cytokines and decrease the level of BDNF, they are detrimental to the developing fetus.

Poor sleep quality has been associated with:

- A 1.25 times increased risk of preterm birth

Sleep duration lasting less than 8 hours per night has been associated with:

- A 3.80 times higher risk of miscarriage during the first and second trimester

- A 2.84 times higher risk of low birth weight

However, it has to be noted that the sleep duration here was based on maternal subjective report, and research suggests that pregnant women actually sleep about 30 minutes less than they subjectively report.

64. What if I snore?

Habitual snorers are at risk for sleep disorders, such as obstructive sleep apnea. Snoring causes sleep deprivation and daytime sleepiness. Maternal snoring during pregnancy has been linked to a higher risk of preterm birth, low birth weight, and fetal growth restriction.

If you snore frequently, you had better seek help from a doctor.

65. Am I sleeping well?

You can take a sleep quality test at https://brainandlife.net/test-sleep-quality to answer this question.

A total score ≤ 5 indicates good sleep quality while a total score > 5 indicates poor sleep quality. If you score >5, read the following item 66 How can I improve sleep quality carefully to ensure a healthy habit of sleep and refer to a doctor if necessary.

66. How can I improve sleep quality?

Obtaining enough sleep day-to-day obviously is important, but obtaining high-quality sleep is essential as well. A dozen specific strategies that help optimize sleep are presented below:

- Establish more regularity and consistency in the timing of daily activities, especially the timing of getting up, evening meals, and bedtime routine. For example, you may want to read, take a hot shower, and then go to bed. Higher levels of regularity in behavioral rhythms are associated with better sleep outcomes, lower depression, and improved health.

- Make your bedroom quiet, cool, and dark, and your bed comfortable to promote sleep.

- Use your bedroom only for sleep, do not work or watch TV or videos in bed. This helps to establish a conditioning between your bedroom and sleep.

- Nap early, keep it short and before 5 p.m. Regular napping has been associated with enhanced mood, reduced risk of cardiovascular diseases and better cognitive functioning; but late napping may interfere with night sleep.

- Avoid caffeine, alcohol, and nicotine for three to six hours before bedtime, as these chemicals interfere with sleep; not only this, avoid them at all because they are toxic to your baby.

- Avoid heavy meals 2–3 hours before bedtime. Eating big or spicy meals may cause discomfort and interfere with sleep. If you feel hungry, try a light snack at least 45 minutes before bedtime.

- Consume enough drinks during the day, but balance it before sleep so that you won't wake up thirsty nor have to go to bathroom in the middle of sleep.

- Do not use light-emitting electronic devices such as cell phones and tablets before bedtime, as it has negative effects on sleep.

- Exercise every day, as regular exercise improves sleep quality. But try to avoid vigorous exercise within 2 hours of going to bed, for vigorous late-night exercise may produce increased arousal and prolong your sleep onset latency.

- Try to reduce total sitting time and time spent television viewing. The more total sitting time and time spent viewing television, the greater odds of long sleep onset latency ($\geq$ 30 min), waking up too early in the morning and poor sleep quality, and the higher risk for obstructive sleep apnea.

- If you can't fall asleep after 20–30 minutes, get out of bed, go to another room, and do something relaxing, for example reading or listening to slow, soothing music until you are tired enough to sleep.

- Don't stare at your clock at night. It actually increases stress and interferes with sleep.

POSTSCRIPT

I hope you have seen how your health and behavior, no matter how subtle it may seem to you, have a powerful and long-lasting impact on your baby's developing brain. Your nutritional status and lifestyle are the seed of your baby's intelligence. Why not optimize that seed and make it a gift to your future, precious baby?

If you want to learn more about the optimal lifestyle during pregnancy, sign up to my newsletters at http://brainandlife.net and follow me on twitter @ChongChenBlog, I will share more research digests with you. You can also write to me at chen@brainandlife.net to ask questions.

If you enjoyed this book, please leave a brief review on Amazon or Goodreads to let more people discover it. Thanks.

REFERENCES

Quote: Janet DiPietro… Janet L. Hopson. (Sep/Oct 1998). Fetal Psychology: Your baby can feel, dream and even listen to Mozart in the womb. Psychology Today. Available at https://www.psychologytoday.com/articles/199809/fetal-psychology (last accessed 2017/08/10)

PART 1: THE SEED OF INTELLIGENCE

1. Your baby experiences a remarkable rate of development in the womb

Stiles, J., & Jernigan, T. L. (2010). The basics of brain development. *Neuropsychology review*, *20*(4), 327-348.

DiPietro, J.A. Prenatal Development. (2008) M. Haith and J. Benson (Eds), *Encyclopedia of Infant and Early Childhood Development*. Volume 2, pp 604-614. San Diego: Elsevier, Inc.

Cowan, W. M. (1979). The development of the brain. *Scientific American*, *241*(3), 113-133.

Levitt, P. (2003). Structural and functional maturation of the developing primate brain. *The Journal of pediatrics*, *143*(4), 35-45.

2. The seed of intelligence dissected

National Health and Medical Research Council. *Healthy Eating During Your Pregnancy: Advice on Eating for you and Your Baby*. Canberra ACT, Australia: Department of Health and Ageing, 2014.

Kodomari, I., Wada, E., Nakamura, S., & Wada, K. (2009). Maternal supply of BDNF to mouse fetal brain through the placenta. *Neurochemistry international, 54*(2), 95-98.

Park, H., & Poo, M. M. (2013). Neurotrophin regulation of neural circuit development and function. *Nature Reviews Neuroscience, 14*(1), 7-23.

Chen, C. (2017). *Plato's Insight: How Physical Exercise Boosts Mental Excellence.* London: Brain & Life Publishing

Baskin, R., Hill, B., Jacka, F. N., O'Neil, A., & Skouteris, H. (2015). The association between diet quality and mental health during the perinatal period. A systematic review. *Appetite, 91*, 41-47.

Emmett, P. M., Jones, L. R., & Golding, J. (2015). Pregnancy diet and associated outcomes in the Avon Longitudinal Study of Parents and Children. *Nutrition reviews, 73*(suppl_3), 154-174.

Shivappa, N., Steck, S. E., Hurley, T. G., Hussey, J. R., & Hébert, J. R. (2014). Designing and developing a literature-derived, population-based dietary inflammatory index. *Public health nutrition*, 17(8), 1689-1696.

Ekdahl, C. T., Claasen, J. H., Bonde, S., Kokaia, Z., & Lindvall, O. (2003). Inflammation is detrimental for neurogenesis in adult brain. *Proceedings of the National Academy of Sciences, 100*(23), 13632-13637.

Gorelick, P. B. (2010). Role of inflammation in cognitive impairment: results of observational epidemiological studies and clinical trials. *Annals of the New York Academy of Sciences, 1207*(1), 155-162.

Dantzer, R., O'Connor, J. C., Freund, G. G., Johnson, R. W., & Kelley, K. W. (2008). From inflammation to sickness and depression: when the immune system subjugates the brain. *Nature reviews. Neuroscience*, 9(1), 46.

Amarilyo, G., Oren, A., Mimouni, F. B., Ochshorn, Y., Deutsch, V., & Mandel, D. (2011). Increased cord serum inflammatory markers in small-for-gestational-age neonates. *Journal of Perinatology*, 31(1), 30.

Ernst, G. D., de Jonge, L. L., Hofman, A., Lindemans, J., Russcher, H., Steegers, E. A., & Jaddoe, V. W. (2011). C-reactive protein levels in early pregnancy, fetal growth patterns, and the risk for neonatal complications: the Generation R Study. *American journal of obstetrics and gynecology*, 205(2), 132-e1.

Scholl, T. O., Chen, X., Goldberg, G. S., Khusial, P. R., & Stein, T. P. (2011). Maternal diet, C-reactive protein, and the outcome of pregnancy. *Journal of the American College of Nutrition*, 30(4), 233-240.

3. Why pregnancy provides a perfect opportunity for health revolution?

Anderson, A. S. (2001). Pregnancy as a time for dietary change?. *Proceedings of the nutrition society*, 60(4), 497-504.

Kemmer, D., Anderson, A. S., & Marshall, D. W. (1998). Living together and eating together: changes in food choice and eating habits during the transition from single to married/cohabiting. *The Sociological Review*, 46(1), 48-72.

McLeod, E. R., Campbell, K. J., & Hesketh, K. D. (2011). Nutrition knowledge: a mediator between socioeconomic position and diet quality in Australian first-time mothers. *Journal of the American Dietetic Association, 111*(5), 696-704.

Szwajcer, E. M., Hiddink, G. J., Koelen, M. A., & Van Woerkum, C. M. J. (2005). Nutrition-related information-seeking behaviours before and throughout the course of pregnancy: consequences for nutrition communication. *European Journal of Clinical Nutrition, 59*, S57-S65.

4. Many people make changes during pregnancy, but most lack adequate knowledge on a healthy lifestyle

Hillier, S. E., & Olander, E. K. (2017). Women's dietary changes before and during pregnancy: A systematic review. *Midwifery*.

NHaMR, C. (2003). Dietary Guidelines for Children and Adolescents in Australia incorporating the Infant Feeding Guidelines for Health Workers. *Canberra: Commonwealth of Australia*.

Wilkinson, S. A., Miller, Y. D., & Watson, B. (2009). Prevalence of health behaviours in pregnancy at service entry in a Queensland health service district. *Australian and New Zealand Journal of Public Health, 33*(3), 228-233.

Tong, V. T., England, L. J., Dietz, P. M., & Asare, L. A. (2008). Smoking patterns and use of cessation interventions during pregnancy. *American journal of preventive medicine, 35*(4), 327-333.

Tong, V. T., Dietz, P. M., Farr, S. L., D'angelo, D. V., & England, L. J. (2013). Estimates of smoking before and during pregnancy, and smoking cessation during pregnancy: comparing two population-based data sources. *Public health reports*, *128*(3), 179-188.

Mparmpakas, D., Goumenou, A., Zachariades, E., Pados, G., Gidron, Y., & Karteris, E. (2013). Immune system function, stress, exercise and nutrition profile can affect pregnancy outcome: lessons from a Mediterranean cohort. *Experimental and therapeutic medicine*, *5*(2), 411-418.

Paulik, E., Császár, J., Kozinszky, Z., & Nagymajtényi, L. (2009). Preconceptional and prenatal predictors of folic acid intake in Hungarian pregnant women. *European Journal of Obstetrics & Gynecology and Reproductive Biology*, *145*(1), 49-52.

de Jersey, S. J., Nicholson, J. M., Callaway, L. K., & Daniels, L. A. (2013). An observational study of nutrition and physical activity behaviours, knowledge, and advice in pregnancy. *BMC pregnancy and childbirth*, *13*(1), 115.

Takimoto, H., Mitsuishi, C., & Kato, N. (2011). Attitudes toward pregnancy related changes and self-judged dieting behavior. *Asia Pacific journal of clinical nutrition*, *20*(2), 212-219.

Phelan, S. (2010). Pregnancy: a "teachable moment" for weight control and obesity prevention. *American journal of obstetrics and gynecology*, *202*(2), 135-e1.

Black, R. E., Allen, L. H., Bhutta, Z. A., Caulfield, L. E., De Onis, M., Ezzati, M., ... & Maternal and Child Undernutrition Study Group. (2008). Maternal and child undernutrition: global and regional exposures and health consequences. *The lancet*, *371*(9608), 243-260.

Victora, C. G., Adair, L., Fall, C., Hallal, P. C., Martorell, R., Richter, L., ... & Maternal and Child Undernutrition Study Group. (2008). Maternal and child undernutrition: consequences for adult health and human capital. *The lancet*, *371*(9609), 340-357.

5. Why is unplanned pregnancy dangerous?

Department of Health (2000) *Folic Acid and the Prevention of Disease. Report of the Committee on Medical Aspects of Food Policy*. London: H.M. Stationery Office

Flower, A., Shawe, J., Stephenson, J., & Doyle, P. (2013). Pregnancy planning, smoking behaviour during pregnancy, and neonatal outcome: UK Millennium Cohort Study. *BMC pregnancy and childbirth*, 13(1), 238.

May, P. A., Baete, A., Russo, J., Elliott, A. J., Blankenship, J., Kalberg, W. O., ... & Adam, M. P. (2014). Prevalence and characteristics of fetal alcohol spectrum disorders. *Pediatrics*, 134(5), 855-866.

Miller, L. J., & LaRusso, E. M. (2011). Preventing postpartum depression. *Psychiatric Clinics of North America*, 34(1), 53-65.

Keen, C. L., Uriu-Adams, J. Y., Skalny, A., Grabeklis, A., Grabeklis, S., Green, K., ... & Chambers, C. D. (2010). The plausibility of maternal nutritional status being a contributing factor to the risk for fetal alcohol spectrum disorders: the potential influence of zinc status as an example. *Biofactors*, 36(2), 125-135.

6. Concerns for single mothers

Shah, P. S., Zao, J., & Ali, S. (2011). Maternal marital status and birth outcomes: a systematic review and meta-analyses. *Maternal and child health journal, 15*(7), 1097-1109.

Elfhag, K., & Rasmussen, F. (2008). Food consumption, eating behaviour and self-esteem among single v. married and cohabiting mothers and their 12-year-old children. *Public health nutrition, 11*(9), 934-939.

Northstone, K., Emmett, P., & Rogers, I. (2008). Dietary patterns in pregnancy and associations with socio-demographic and lifestyle factors. *European Journal of Clinical Nutrition, 62*(4), 471.

Farbu, J., Haugen, M., Meltzer, H. M., & Brantsæter, A. L. (2014). Impact of singlehood during pregnancy on dietary intake and birth outcomes-a study in the Norwegian Mother and Child Cohort Study. *BMC pregnancy and childbirth*, 14(1), 396.

Henriksen, R. E., Torsheim, T., & Thuen, F. (2014). Loneliness, social integration and consumption of sugar-containing beverages: testing the social baseline theory. *PloS one, 9*(8), e104421.

7. I'm giving birth in rapid succession or to twins, what should I be wary of?

Houwelingen, A. C., & Hornstra, G. (1997). Relation between birth order and the maternal and neonatal DHA status. *The European Journal of Clinical Nutrition, 51*(8), 548-553.

Al, M. D., Hornstra, G., van der Schouw, Y. T., Bulstra-Ramakers, M. T., & Huisjes, H. J. (1990). Biochemical EFA status of mothers and their neonates after normal pregnancy. *Early human development, 24*(3), 239-248.

Holley, W. L., Rosenbaum, A. L., & Churchill, J. A. (1969). Effect of rapid succession of pregnancy. In: Pan American Health Organization. *Perinatal factors affecting human development* (pp. 41-44). Washington, D.C.

8. How often should I attend antenatal care during pregnancy?

World Health Organization. (2006). *Provision of effective antenatal care: integrated management of pregnancy and childbirth (IMPAC)*. Geneva: Standards for maternal and neonatal care (1.6), Department of making pregnancy safer.

World Health Organization. (2009). *WHO recommended interventions for improving maternal and newborn health: integrated management of pregnancy and childbirth*. Geneva: World Health Organization.

Kattula, D., Sarkar, R., Sivarathinaswamy, P., Velusamy, V., Venugopal, S., Naumova, E. N., ... & Kang, G. (2014). The first 1000 days of life: prenatal and postnatal risk factors for morbidity and growth in a birth cohort in southern India. *BMJ open*, *4*(7), e005404.

World health Organization. (2016). *WHO recommendations on antenatal care for a positive pregnancy experience*. Geneva: World Health Organization.

PART 2: DIET & NUTRITION

9. How does maternal undernutrition affect the baby? Lessons from the 1944-1945 Dutch Famine and the 1959-1961 Chinese Famine

Painter, R. C., Roseboom, T. J., & Bleker, O. P. (2005). Prenatal exposure to the Dutch famine and disease in later life: an overview. *Reproductive toxicology*, *20*(3), 345-352.

Schulz, L. C. (2010). The Dutch Hunger Winter and the developmental origins of health and disease. *Proceedings of the National Academy of Sciences*, *107*(39), 16757-16758.

Roseboom, T., de Rooij, S., & Painter, R. (2006). The Dutch famine and its long-term consequences for adult health. *Early human development*, *82*(8), 485-491.

Franzek, E. J., Sprangers, N., Janssens, A. C. J. W., Van Duijn, C. M., & Van De Wetering, B. J. (2008). Prenatal exposure to the 1944–45 Dutch 'hunger winter' and addiction later in life. *Addiction*, *103*(3), 433-438.

Brown, A. S., Susser, E. S., Lin, S. P., Neugebauer, R., & Gorman, J. M. (1995). Increased risk of affective disorders in males after second trimester prenatal exposure to the Dutch hunger winter of 1944-45. *The British Journal of Psychiatry*, *166*(5), 601-606.

Brown, A. S., van Os, J., Driessens, C., Hoek, H. W., & Susser, E. S. (2000). Further evidence of relation between prenatal famine and major affective disorder. *American Journal of Psychiatry*, *157*(2), 190-195.

de Rooij, S. R., Wouters, H., Yonker, J. E., Painter, R. C., & Roseboom, T. J. (2010). Prenatal undernutrition and cognitive function in late adulthood. *Proceedings of the National Academy of Sciences*, *107*(39), 16881-16886.

Li, J., Na, L., Ma, H., Zhang, Z., Li, T., Lin, L., ... & Li, Y. (2015). Multigenerational effects of parental prenatal exposure to famine on adult offspring cognitive function. *Scientific reports*, *5*.

St Clair, D., Xu, M., Wang, P., Yu, Y., Fang, Y., Zhang, F., ... & He, L. (2005). Rates of adult schizophrenia following prenatal exposure to the Chinese famine of 1959-1961. *Jama*, *294*(5), 557-562.

10. What if I'm very thin?

Fishman SM, Caulfield L, de Onis M, et al. Childhood and maternal underweight. In: Ezzati M, Lopez AD, Rodgers A, Murray CLJ, eds. *Comparative quantification of health risks: global and regional burden of disease attributable to selected major risk factors*. Geneva: World Health Organization, 2004: 39–161.

Yanney, M., & Marlow, N. (2004, October). Paediatric consequences of fetal growth restriction. In *Seminars in Fetal and Neonatal Medicine* (Vol. 9, No. 5, pp. 411-418). WB Saunders.

Barker, D. J. (2006). Adult consequences of fetal growth restriction. *Clinical obstetrics and gynecology*, *49*(2), 270-283.

Han, Z., Mulla, S., Beyene, J., Liao, G., & McDonald, S. D. (2010). Maternal underweight and the risk of preterm birth and low birth weight: a systematic review and meta-analyses. *International journal of epidemiology*, *40*(1), 65-101.

Helgstrand, S., & Andersen, A. M. N. (2005). Maternal underweight and the risk of spontaneous abortion. *Acta obstetricia et gynecologica Scandinavica*, *84*(12), 1197-1201.

Black, R. E., Allen, L. H., Bhutta, Z. A., Caulfield, L. E., De Onis, M., Ezzati, M., ... & Maternal and Child Undernutrition Study Group. (2008). Maternal and child undernutrition: global and regional exposures and health consequences. *The lancet*, *371*(9608), 243-260.

Polańska, K., Muszyński, P., Sobala, W., Dziewirska, E., Merecz-Kot, D., & Hanke, W. (2015). Maternal lifestyle during pregnancy and child psychomotor development—Polish Mother and Child Cohort study. *Early human development*, *91*(5), 317-325.

Mangili, A., Murman, D. H., Zampini, A. M., Wanke, C. A., & Mayer, K. H. (2006). Nutrition and HIV infection: review of weight loss and wasting in the era of highly active antiretroviral therapy from the nutrition for healthy living cohort. *Clinical Infectious Diseases*, *42*(6), 836-842.

11. Can I diet while pregnant?

National Institute of Health and Clinical Excellence. (2010). *Weight management before, during and after pregnancy*

Hytten, F.E. (1983) Nutritional physiology during pregnancy. In *Nutrition in Pregnancy* pp. 1–18 [DM Campbell and DG Gillmer, editors]. London: Royal College of Gynaecologists

Takimoto, H., Mitsuishi, C., & Kato, N. (2011). Attitudes toward pregnancy related changes and self-judged dieting behavior. *Asia Pacific journal of clinical nutrition*, *20*(2), 212-219.

Black, R. E., Allen, L. H., Bhutta, Z. A., Caulfield, L. E., De Onis, M., Ezzati, M., ... & Maternal and Child Undernutrition Study Group. (2008). Maternal and child undernutrition: global and regional exposures and health consequences. *The lancet*, *371*(9608), 243-260.

Victora, C. G., Adair, L., Fall, C., Hallal, P. C., Martorell, R., Richter, L., ... & Maternal and Child Undernutrition Study Group. (2008). Maternal and child undernutrition: consequences for adult health and human capital. *The lancet*, *371*(9609), 340-357.

Schlotz, W., & Phillips, D. I. (2009). Fetal origins of mental health: evidence and mechanisms. *Brain, behavior, and immunity*, *23*(7), 905-916.

Rodriguez, J. S., Bartlett, T. Q., Keenan, K. E., Nathanielsz, P. W., & Nijland, M. J. (2012). Sex-dependent cognitive performance in baboon offspring following maternal caloric restriction in pregnancy and lactation. *Reproductive sciences*, *19*(5), 493-504.

Reyes-Castro, L. A., Rodriguez, J. S., Rodriguez-Gonzalez, G. L., Chavira, R., Bautista, C. J., McDonald, T. J., ... & Zambrano, E. (2012). Pre-and/or postnatal protein restriction developmentally programs affect and risk assessment behaviors in adult male rats. *Behavioural brain research*, *227*(2), 324-329.

12. Why shouldn't I skip meals?

Institute of Medicine (US). Subcommittee for a Clinical Application Guide. (1992). *Nutrition During Pregnancy and Lactation:: An Implementation Guide*. National Academies.

Maria Siega-Riz, A., Herrmann, T. S., Savitz, D. A., & Thorp, J. M. (2001). Frequency of eating during pregnancy and its effect on preterm delivery. *American journal of epidemiology*, *153*(7), 647-652.

13. Are vegan-vegetarian diets dangerous during pregnancy?

Piccoli, G. B., Clari, R., Vigotti, F. N., Leone, F., Attini, R., Cabiddu, G., ... & Pani, A. (2015). Vegan-vegetarian diets in pregnancy: danger or panacea? A systematic narrative review. *BJOG: An International Journal of Obstetrics & Gynaecology*, 122(5), 623-633.

Craig, W. J., & Mangels, A. R. (2009). Position of the American Dietetic Association: vegetarian diets. *Journal of the American Dietetic Association*, *109*(7), 1266-1282.

14. How much extra energy intake do I need?

U.S. Institute of Medicine. (2006) *Dietary Reference Intakes, The Essential Guide to Nutrient Requirements*. Washington DC: National Academies Press

U.K. National Institute for Health and Care Excellence (2010). Weight management before, during and after pregnancy. https://www.nice.org.uk/guidance/ph27 (last accessed 2017/8/10)

US Department of Health and Human Services. (2015). *2015–2020 dietary guidelines for Americans*. Washington (DC): USDA.

Hercberg, S. *Prenatal Nutrition Guidelines for Health Professionals-Iron contributes to a healthy pregnancy. Majesty the Queen in Right of Canada, represented by the Minister of Health Canada 2009. ISBN: 978-1-100-12207-6 (PDF Version) Cat. No*. H164-109/1-2009E-PDF.

15. What is the most recommended healthy diet?

Kushi, L. H., Lenart, E. B., & Willett, W. C. (1995). Health implications of Mediterranean diets in light of contemporary knowledge. 1. Plant foods and dairy products. *The American journal of clinical nutrition, 61*(6), 1407S-1415S.

Kushi, L. H., Lenart, E. B., & Willett, W. C. (1995). Health implications of Mediterranean diets in light of contemporary knowledge. 2. Meat, wine, fats, and oils. *The American journal of clinical nutrition, 61*(6), 1416S-1427S.

Rao, J. S., Ertley, R. N., Lee, H. J., DeMar Jr, J. C., Arnold, J. T., Rapoport, S. I., & Bazinet, R. P. (2007). n-3 polyunsaturated fatty acid deprivation in rats decreases frontal cortex BDNF via a p38 MAPK-dependent mechanism. *Molecular psychiatry, 12*(1), 36.

Wu, A., Ying, Z., & Gomez-Pinilla, F. (2008). Docosahexaenoic acid dietary supplementation enhances the effects of exercise on synaptic plasticity and cognition. *Neuroscience, 155*(3), 751-759.

Hadjighassem, M., Kamalidehghan, B., Shekarriz, N., Baseerat, A., Molavi, N., Mehrpour, M., ... & Meng, G. Y. (2015). Oral consumption of α-linolenic acid increases serum BDNF levels in healthy adult humans. *Nutrition journal, 14*(1), 20.

Beltz, B. S., Tlusty, M. F., Benton, J. L., & Sandeman, D. C. (2007). Omega-3 fatty acids upregulate adult neurogenesis. *Neuroscience letters, 415*(2), 154-158.

Esmaillzadeh, A., Kimiagar, M., Mehrabi, Y., Azadbakht, L., Hu, F. B., & Willett, W. C. (2006). Fruit and vegetable intakes, C-reactive protein, and the metabolic syndrome. *The American journal of clinical nutrition, 84*(6), 1489-1497.

Wannamethee, S. G., Lowe, G. D., Rumley, A., Bruckdorfer, K. R., & Whincup, P. H. (2006). Associations of vitamin C status, fruit and vegetable intakes, and markers of inflammation and hemostasis. *The American journal of clinical nutrition*, *83*(3), 567-574.

Gonzalez, R., Ballester, I., López-Posadas, R., Suárez, M. D., Zarzuelo, A., Martinez-Augustin, O., & Medina, F. S. D. (2011). Effects of flavonoids and other polyphenols on inflammation. *Critical reviews in food science and nutrition*, *51*(4), 331-362.

Andre, C. M., Greenwood, J. M., Walker, E. G., Rassam, M., Sullivan, M., Evers, D., ... & Laing, W. A. (2012). Anti-inflammatory procyanidins and triterpenes in 109 apple varieties. *Journal of agricultural and food chemistry*, *60*(42), 10546-10554.

Coelho, R. C. L. A., Hermsdorff, H. H. M., & Bressan, J. (2013). Anti-inflammatory properties of orange juice: possible favorable molecular and metabolic effects. *Plant foods for human nutrition*, *68*(1), 1-10.

Ismail, T., Sestili, P., & Akhtar, S. (2012). Pomegranate peel and fruit extracts: a review of potential anti-inflammatory and anti-infective effects. *Journal of ethnopharmacology*, *143*(2), 397-405.

Chrysohoou, C., Panagiotakos, D. B., Pitsavos, C., Das, U. N., & Stefanadis, C. (2004). Adherence to the Mediterranean diet attenuates inflammation and coagulation process in healthy adults: The ATTICA Study. *Journal of the American College of Cardiology*, *44*(1), 152-158.

Esposito, K., Marfella, R., Ciotola, M., Di Palo, C., Giugliano, F., Giugliano, G., ... & Giugliano, D. (2004). Effect of a Mediterranean-style diet on endothelial dysfunction and markers of vascular inflammation in the metabolic syndrome: a randomized trial. *Jama*, *292*(12), 1440-1446.

Timmermans, S., Steegers-Theunissen, R. P., Vujkovic, M., Bakker, R., den Breeijen, H., Raat, H., ... & Steegers, E. A. (2011). Major dietary patterns and blood pressure patterns during pregnancy: the Generation R Study. *American journal of obstetrics and gynecology, 205*(4), 337-e1.

Khoury, J., Henriksen, T., Christophersen, B., & Tonstad, S. (2005). Effect of a cholesterol-lowering diet on maternal, cord, and neonatal lipids, and pregnancy outcome: a randomized clinical trial. *American journal of obstetrics and gynecology, 193*(4), 1292-1301.

Hirai, S., Takahashi, N., Goto, T., Lin, S., Uemura, T., Yu, R., & Kawada, T. (2010). Functional food targeting the regulation of obesity-induced inflammatory responses and pathologies. *Mediators of inflammation, 2010*.

Baskin, R., Hill, B., Jacka, F. N., O'Neil, A., & Skouteris, H. (2015). The association between diet quality and mental health during the perinatal period. A systematic review. *Appetite, 91*, 41-47.

Steenweg-de Graaff, J., Tiemeier, H., Steegers-Theunissen, R. P., Hofman, A., Jaddoe, V. W., Verhulst, F. C., & Roza, S. J. (2014). Maternal dietary patterns during pregnancy and child internalising and externalising problems. The Generation R Study. *Clinical nutrition, 33*(1), 115-121.

Jacka, F. N., Ystrom, E., Brantsaeter, A. L., Karevold, E., Roth, C., Haugen, M., ... & Berk, M. (2013). Maternal and early postnatal nutrition and mental health of offspring by age 5 years: a prospective cohort study. *Journal of the American Academy of Child & Adolescent Psychiatry*, 52(10), 1038-1047.

16. Why should I eat fruits and vegetables daily?

Polidori, M. C., Praticó, D., Mangialasche, F., Mariani, E., Aust, O., Anlasik, T., ... & Mecocci, P. (2009). High fruit and vegetable intake is positively correlated with antioxidant status and cognitive performance in healthy subjects. *Journal of Alzheimer's Disease*, *17*(4), 921-927.

Péneau, S., Galan, P., Jeandel, C., Ferry, M., Andreeva, V., Hercberg, S., ... & SU. VI. MAX 2 Research Group. (2011). Fruit and vegetable intake and cognitive function in the SU. VI. MAX 2 prospective study. *The American journal of clinical nutrition*, *94*(5), 1295-1303.

Hung, H. C., Joshipura, K. J., Jiang, R., Hu, F. B., Hunter, D., Smith-Warner, S. A., ... & Willett, W. C. (2004). Fruit and vegetable intake and risk of major chronic disease. *Journal of the National Cancer Institute*, *96*(21), 1577-1584.

Tobias, M., Turley, M., Stefanogiannis, N., Hoorn, S. V., Lawes, C., Mhurchu, C. N., & Rodgers, A. (2006). Vegetable and fruit intake and mortality from chronic disease in New Zealand. *Australian and New Zealand journal of public health*, *30*(1), 26-31.

Bolduc, F. V., Lau, A., Rosenfelt, C. S., Langer, S., Wang, N., Smithson, L., ... & Becker, A. B. (2016). Cognitive enhancement in infants associated with increased maternal fruit intake during pregnancy: results from a birth cohort study with validation in an animal model. *EBioMedicine*, 8, 331-340.

Mennella, J. A., & Beauchamp, G. K. (1991). Maternal diet alters the sensory qualities of human milk and the nursling's behavior. *Pediatrics*, *88*(4), 737-744.

Emmett, P. M., Jones, L. R., & Golding, J. (2015). Pregnancy diet and associated outcomes in the Avon Longitudinal Study of Parents and Children. *Nutrition reviews*, *73*(suppl_3), 154-174.

17. How much fruit should I eat daily?

U.S. Department of Agriculture. *All About the Fruit Group.* https://www.choosemyplate.gov/fruit (last accessed 2017/8/10)

US Department of Health and Human Services. (2015). *2015–2020 dietary guidelines for Americans*. Washington (DC): USDA.

Bolduc, F. V., Lau, A., Rosenfelt, C. S., Langer, S., Wang, N., Smithson, L., ... & Becker, A. B. (2016). Cognitive enhancement in infants associated with increased maternal fruit intake during pregnancy: results from a birth cohort study with validation in an animal model. *EBioMedicine*, 8, 331-340.

18. How many vegetables should I eat daily?

U.S. Department of Agriculture. *All about the Vegetable Group.* https://www.choosemyplate.gov/vegetables (last accessed 2017/8/10)

US Department of Health and Human Services. (2015). *2015–2020 dietary guidelines for Americans*. Washington (DC): USDA.

19. How much and what kind of protein should I consume daily?

US Department of Health and Human Services. (2015). *2015–2020 dietary guidelines for Americans*. Washington (DC): USDA.

U.S. Department of Agriculture. *All about the Protein Foods Group*. https://www.choosemyplate.gov/protein-foods (last accessed 2017/8/10)

20. Why should I eat seafood regularly?

Morris, M. C., Evans, D. A., Bienias, J. L., Tangney, C. C., Bennett, D. A., Wilson, R. S., ... & Schneider, J. (2003). Consumption of fish and n-3 fatty acids and risk of incident Alzheimer disease. *Archives of neurology*, *60*(7), 940-946.

Kris-Etherton, P. M., Harris, W. S., & Appel, L. J. (2002). Fish consumption, fish oil, omega-3 fatty acids, and cardiovascular disease. *circulation*, *106*(21), 2747-2757.

Emmett, P. M., Jones, L. R., & Golding, J. (2015). Pregnancy diet and associated outcomes in the Avon Longitudinal Study of Parents and Children. *Nutrition reviews*, *73*(suppl_3), 154-174.

Sagiv, S. K., Thurston, S. W., Bellinger, D. C., Amarasiriwardena, C., & Korrick, S. A. (2012). Prenatal exposure to mercury and fish consumption during pregnancy and attention-deficit/hyperactivity disorder–related behavior in children. *Archives of pediatrics & adolescent medicine*, *166*(12), 1123-1131.

21. Seafood may be contaminated by mercury, should I still eat it frequently?

World Health Organization. (2007). Exposure to mercury: A major public health concern. *WHO, Public Health and Environment*.

Debes, F., Budtz-Jørgensen, E., Weihe, P., White, R. F., & Grandjean, P. (2006). Impact of prenatal methylmercury exposure on neurobehavioral function at age 14 years. *Neurotoxicology and teratology*, *28*(3), 363-375.

Llop, S., Guxens, M., Murcia, M., Lertxundi, A., Ramon, R., Riaño, I., ... & Ballester, F. (2012). Prenatal exposure to mercury and infant neurodevelopment in a multicenter cohort in Spain: study of potential modifiers. *American journal of epidemiology*, *175*(5), 451-465.

Deroma, L., Parpinel, M., Tognin, V., Channoufi, L., Tratnik, J., Horvat, M., ... & Barbone, F. (2013). Neuropsychological assessment at school-age and prenatal low-level exposure to mercury through fish consumption in an Italian birth cohort living near a contaminated site. *International journal of hygiene and environmental health*, *216*(4), 486-493.

Oken, E., Radesky, J. S., Wright, R. O., Bellinger, D. C., Amarasiriwardena, C. J., Kleinman, K. P., ... & Gillman, M. W. (2008). Maternal fish intake during pregnancy, blood mercury levels, and child cognition at age 3 years in a US cohort. *American journal of epidemiology*, *167*(10), 1171-1181.

Sagiv, S. K., Thurston, S. W., Bellinger, D. C., Amarasiriwardena, C., & Korrick, S. A. (2012). Prenatal exposure to mercury and fish consumption during pregnancy and attention-deficit/hyperactivity disorder–related behavior in children. *Archives of pediatrics & adolescent medicine*, *166*(12), 1123-1131.

EPA website, *Fish Consumption Advisories, General Information*. Available at:

http://water.epa.gov/scitech/swguidance/fishshellfish/fishadvisori
es/general.cfm (last accessed 2017/8/10)

22. Can I eat canned seafood?

Deroma, L., Parpinel, M., Tognin, V., Channoufi, L., Tratnik, J., Horvat, M., ... & Barbone, F. (2013). Neuropsychological assessment at school-age and prenatal low-level exposure to mercury through fish consumption in an Italian birth cohort living near a contaminated site. *International journal of hygiene and environmental health, 216*(4), 486-493.

Castro-González, M. I., & Méndez-Armenta, M. (2008). Heavy metals: Implications associated to fish consumption. *Environmental toxicology and pharmacology, 26*(3), 263-271.

US Department of Health and Human Services. (2015). *2015– 2020 dietary guidelines for Americans.* Washington (DC): USDA.

Aubourg, S. P. (2001). Loss of quality during the manufacture of canned fish products. *Revista de Agaroquimica y Tecnologia de Alimentos, 7*(3), 199-215.

23. How much and what kind of seafood should I eat per week?

US Department of Health and Human Services. (2015). *2015– 2020 dietary guidelines for Americans.* Washington (DC): USDA.

EPA website, *Fish Consumption Advisories, General Information.* Available at: http://water.epa.gov/scitech/swguidance/fishshellfish/fishadvisori es/general.cfm (last accessed 2017/8/10)

24. Why should I consume dairy?

Miller, G. D., Jarvis, J. K., & McBean, L. D. (2006). *Handbook of dairy foods and nutrition*. CRC press.

Miller, G. D., DiRienzo, D. D., Reusser, M. E., & McCarron, D. A. (2000). Benefits of dairy product consumption on blood pressure in humans: a summary of the biomedical literature. *Journal of the american College of Nutrition, 19*(sup2), 147S-164S.

Davoodi, H., Esmaeili, S., & Mortazavian, A. M. (2013). Effects of milk and milk products consumption on cancer: a review. *Comprehensive Reviews in Food Science and Food Safety, 12*(3), 249-264.

Malik, V. S., Sun, Q., van Dam, R. M., Rimm, E. B., Willett, W. C., Rosner, B., & Hu, F. B. (2011). Adolescent dairy product consumption and risk of type 2 diabetes in middle-aged women. *The American journal of clinical nutrition*, ajcn-009621.

Miyake, Y., Tanaka, K., Okubo, H., Sasaki, S., & Arakawa, M. (2015). Intake of dairy products and calcium and prevalence of depressive symptoms during pregnancy in Japan: a cross-sectional study. *BJOG: An International Journal of Obstetrics & Gynaecology, 122*(3), 336-343.

U.S. Department of Agriculture. *All about the Dairy Group.* https://www.choosemyplate.gov/dairy (last accessed 2017/8/10)

25. How much and what kind of dairy should I consume everyday?

U.S. Department of Agriculture. *All about the Dairy Group.* https://www.choosemyplate.gov/dairy (last accessed 2017/8/10)

US Department of Health and Human Services. (2015). *2015– 2020 dietary guidelines for Americans*. Washington (DC): USDA.

26. What is the consequence of a "western" diet?

Micha, R., Wallace, S. K., & Mozaffarian, D. (2010). Red and processed meat consumption and risk of incident coronary heart disease, stroke, and diabetes mellitus. *Circulation*, *121*(21), 2271-2283.

Cross, A. J., Leitzmann, M. F., Gail, M. H., Hollenbeck, A. R., Schatzkin, A., & Sinha, R. (2007). A prospective study of red and processed meat intake in relation to cancer risk. *PLoS medicine*, *4*(12), e325.

Schulze, M. B., Manson, J. E., Willett, W. C., & Hu, F. B. (2003). Processed meat intake and incidence of type 2 diabetes in younger and middle-aged women. *Diabetologia*, *46*(11), 1465-1473.

Zhang, C., Schulze, M. B., Solomon, C. G., & Hu, F. B. (2006). A prospective study of dietary patterns, meat intake and the risk of gestational diabetes mellitus. *Diabetologia*, *49*(11), 2604-2613.

Forslund, H. B., Torgerson, J. S., Sjöström, L., & Lindroos, A. K. (2005). Snacking frequency in relation to energy intake and food choices in obese men and women compared to a reference population. *International journal of obesity*, *29*(6), 711.

Jeffery, R. W., & French, S. A. (1998). Epidemic obesity in the United States: are fast foods and television viewing contributing?. *American journal of public health*, *88*(2), 277-280.

Nicklas, T. A., Yang, S. J., Baranowski, T., Zakeri, I., & Berenson, G. (2003). Eating patterns and obesity in children: The

Bogalusa Heart Study. *American journal of preventive medicine*, *25*(1), 9-16.

Baskin, R., Hill, B., Jacka, F. N., O'Neil, A., & Skouteris, H. (2015). The association between diet quality and mental health during the perinatal period. A systematic review. *Appetite*, *91*, 41-47.

Chatzi, L., Melaki, V., Sarri, K., Apostolaki, I., Roumeliotaki, T., Georgiou, V., ... & Kogevinas, M. (2011). Dietary patterns during pregnancy and the risk of postpartum depression: the mother–child 'Rhea'cohort in Crete, Greece. *Public health nutrition*, *14*(9), 1663-1670.

Baskin, R., Hill, B., Jacka, F. N., O'neil, A., & Skouteris, H. (2017). Antenatal dietary patterns and depressive symptoms during pregnancy and early postpartum. *Maternal & child nutrition*, *13*(1).

Jacka, F. N., Ystrom, E., Brantsaeter, A. L., Karevold, E., Roth, C., Haugen, M., ... & Berk, M. (2013). Maternal and early postnatal nutrition and mental health of offspring by age 5 years: a prospective cohort study. *Journal of the American Academy of Child & Adolescent Psychiatry*, 52(10), 1038-1047.

Steenweg-de Graaff, J., Tiemeier, H., Steegers-Theunissen, R. P., Hofman, A., Jaddoe, V. W., Verhulst, F. C., & Roza, S. J. (2014). Maternal dietary patterns during pregnancy and child internalising and externalising problems. The Generation R Study. *Clinical nutrition*, *33*(1), 115-121.

Olafsdottir, A. S., Skuladottir, G. V., Thorsdottir, I., Hauksson, A., & Steingrimsdottir, L. (2006). Maternal diet in early and late pregnancy in relation to weight gain. *International journal of obesity, 30*(3), 492.

Phelan, S., Hart, C., Phipps, M., Abrams, B., Schaffner, A., Adams, A., & Wing, R. (2011). Maternal behaviors during pregnancy impact offspring obesity risk. *Experimental diabetes research, 2011*.

27. What is the consequence of a high-fat diet?

Van Gaal, L. F., Mertens, I. L., & Christophe, E. (2006). Mechanisms linking obesity with cardiovascular disease. *Nature, 444*(7121), 875-880.

Kahn, S. E., Hull, R. L., & Utzschneider, K. M. (2006). Mechanisms linking obesity to insulin resistance and type 2 diabetes. *Nature, 444*(7121), 840.

Frias, A. E., Morgan, T. K., Evans, A. E., Rasanen, J., Oh, K. Y., Thornburg, K. L., & Grove, K. L. (2011). Maternal high-fat diet disturbs uteroplacental hemodynamics and increases the frequency of stillbirth in a nonhuman primate model of excess nutrition. *Endocrinology, 152*(6), 2456-2464.

Sullivan, E. L., Grayson, B., Takahashi, D., Robertson, N., Maier, A., Bethea, C. L., ... & Grove, K. L. (2010). Chronic consumption of a high-fat diet during pregnancy causes perturbations in the serotonergic system and increased anxiety-like behavior in nonhuman primate offspring. *Journal of Neuroscience, 30*(10), 3826-3830.

Sasaki, A., De Vega, W. C., St-Cyr, S., Pan, P., & McGowan, P. O. (2013). Perinatal high fat diet alters glucocorticoid signaling and anxiety behavior in adulthood. *Neuroscience, 240*, 1-12.

Peleg-Raibstein, D., Luca, E., & Wolfrum, C. (2012). Maternal high-fat diet in mice programs emotional behavior in adulthood. *Behavioural brain research, 233*(2), 398-404.

Sullivan, E. L., Nousen, E. K., & Chamlou, K. A. (2014). Maternal high fat diet consumption during the perinatal period programs offspring behavior. *Physiology & behavior, 123*, 236-242.

Yu, H., Bi, Y., Ma, W., He, L., Yuan, L., Feng, J., & Xiao, R. (2010). Long-term effects of high lipid and high energy diet on serum lipid, brain fatty acid composition, and memory and learning ability in mice. *International journal of developmental neuroscience, 28*(3), 271-276.

Ong, Z. Y., & Muhlhausler, B. S. (2011). Maternal "junk-food" feeding of rat dams alters food choices and development of the mesolimbic reward pathway in the offspring. *The FASEB Journal, 25*(7), 2167-2179.

Daenzer, M., Ortmann, S., Klaus, S., & Metges, C. C. (2002). Prenatal high protein exposure decreases energy expenditure and increases adiposity in young rats. *The Journal of nutrition, 132*(2), 142-144.

Vucetic, Z., Kimmel, J., Totoki, K., Hollenbeck, E., & Reyes, T. M. (2010). Maternal high-fat diet alters methylation and gene expression of dopamine and opioid-related genes. *Endocrinology, 151*(10), 4756-4764.

Lu, J., Wu, D. M., Zheng, Y. L., Hu, B., Cheng, W., Zhang, Z. F., & Shan, Q. (2011). Ursolic acid improves high fat diet-induced cognitive impairments by blocking endoplasmic reticulum stress and IκB kinase β/nuclear factor-κB-mediated inflammatory pathways in mice. *Brain, behavior, and immunity*, *25*(8), 1658-1667.

28. Is being obese bad for me?

Chen, C. (2017). *Plato's Insight: How Physical Exercise Boosts Mental Excellence.* London: Brain & Life Publishing

Marchi, J., Berg, M., Dencker, A., Olander, E. K., & Begley, C. (2015). Risks associated with obesity in pregnancy, for the mother and baby: a systematic review of reviews. *Obesity Reviews*, *16*(8), 621-638.

Molyneaux, E., Poston, L., Ashurst-Williams, S., & Howard, L. M. (2014). Obesity and mental disorders during pregnancy and postpartum: a systematic review and meta-analysis. *Obstetrics and gynecology*, *123*(4), 857.

Yu, C. K. H., Teoh, T. G., & Robinson, S. (2006). Obesity in pregnancy. *BJOG: An International Journal of Obstetrics & Gynaecology*, *113*(10), 1117-1125.

Chu, S. Y., Bachman, D. J., Callaghan, W. M., Whitlock, E. P., Dietz, P. M., Berg, C. J., ... & Hornbrook, M. C. (2008). Association between obesity during pregnancy and increased use of health care. *New England Journal of Medicine*, *358*(14), 1444-1453.

29. Is being obese bad for my baby?

Das, U. N. (2001). Is obesity an inflammatory condition?. *Nutrition*, 17(11), 953-966.

Segovia, S. A., Vickers, M. H., Gray, C., & Reynolds, C. M. (2014). Maternal obesity, inflammation, and developmental programming. *BioMed research international*, *2014*.

Stewart, F. M., Freeman, D. J., Ramsay, J. E., Greer, I. A., Caslake, M., & Ferrell, W. R. (2007). Longitudinal assessment of maternal endothelial function and markers of inflammation and placental function throughout pregnancy in lean and obese mothers. *The Journal of Clinical Endocrinology & Metabolism*, *92*(3), 969-975.

Marchi, J., Berg, M., Dencker, A., Olander, E. K., & Begley, C. (2015). Risks associated with obesity in pregnancy, for the mother and baby: a systematic review of reviews. *Obesity Reviews*, *16*(8), 621-638.

Amir, L. H., & Donath, S. (2007). A systematic review of maternal obesity and breastfeeding intention, initiation and duration. *BMC pregnancy and childbirth*, *7*(1), 9.

Rodriguez, A. (2010). Maternal pre-pregnancy obesity and risk for inattention and negative emotionality in children. *Journal of Child Psychology and Psychiatry*, *51*(2), 134-143.

Ray, G. T., Croen, L. A., & Habel, L. A. (2009). Mothers of children diagnosed with attention-deficit/hyperactivity disorder: health conditions and medical care utilization in periods before and after birth of the child. *Medical care*, *47*(1), 105.

30. How much gestational weight gain during pregnancy is healthy and why?

Institute of Medicine. (2009). *Weight Gain During Pregnancy: Re-Examining the Guidelines*. National Academy Press: Washington (DC)

Rasmussen, K. M., Catalano, P. M., & Yaktine, A. L. (2009). New guidelines for weight gain during pregnancy: what obstetrician/gynecologists should know. *Current opinion in obstetrics & gynecology, 21*(6), 521.

Goldstein, R. F., Abell, S. K., Ranasinha, S., Misso, M., Boyle, J. A., Black, M. H., ... & Kim, Y. J. (2017). Association of Gestational Weight Gain With Maternal and Infant Outcomes: A Systematic Review and Meta-analysis. *Jama, 317*(21), 2207-2225.

Cedergren, M. (2006). Effects of gestational weight gain and body mass index on obstetric outcome in Sweden. *International Journal of Gynecology & Obstetrics, 93*(3), 269-274.

Nohr, E. A., Vaeth, M., Baker, J. L., Sørensen, T. I., Olsen, J., & Rasmussen, K. M. (2008). Combined associations of prepregnancy body mass index and gestational weight gain with the outcome of pregnancy. *The American journal of clinical nutrition, 87*(6), 1750-1759.

Rodriguez, A., Miettunen, J., Henriksen, T. B., Olsen, J., Obel, C., Taanila, A., ... & Järvelin, M. R. (2008). Maternal adiposity prior to pregnancy is associated with ADHD symptoms in offspring: evidence from three prospective pregnancy cohorts. *International journal of obesity, 32*(3), 550.

31. How to prevent excessive weight gain during pregnancy?

Muktabhant, B., Lawrie, T. A., Lumbiganon, P., & Laopaiboon, M. (2015). Diet or exercise, or both, for preventing excessive weight gain in pregnancy. *The Cochrane Library*.

De Jersey, S. J., Ross, L. J., Himstedt, K., McIntyre, H. D., & Callaway, L. K. (2011). Weight gain and nutritional intake in obese pregnant women: some clues for intervention. *Nutrition & Dietetics*, *68*(1), 53-59.

Opie, R. S., Neff, M., & Tierney, A. C. (2016). A behavioural nutrition intervention for obese pregnant women: Effects on diet quality, weight gain and the incidence of gestational diabetes. *Australian and New Zealand Journal of Obstetrics and Gynaecology*, *56*(4), 364-373.

Bogaerts, A. F. L., Devlieger, R., Nuyts, E., Witters, I., Gyselaers, W., & Van den Bergh, B. R. H. (2013). Effects of lifestyle intervention in obese pregnant women on gestational weight gain and mental health: a randomized controlled trial. *International Journal of Obesity*, *37*(6), 814-821.

Bogaerts, A. (2014). Obesity and pregnancy, an epidemiological and intervention study from a psychosocial perspective. *Facts, views & vision in ObGyn*, *6*(2), 81.

Jomeen, J. (2004). The importance of assessing psychological status during pregnancy, childbirth and the postnatal period as a multidimensional construct: A literature review. *Clinical Effectiveness in Nursing*, *8*(3), 143-155.

32. What food helps deal with stress and prevent depression?

Rousseau, D., Moreau, D., Raederstorff, D., Sergiel, J. P., Rupp, H., Müggli, R., & Grynberg, A. (1998). Is a dietary n-3 fatty acid supplement able to influence the cardiac effect of the psychological stress?. *Molecular and cellular biochemistry*, *178*(1), 353-366.

Takeuchi, T., Iwanaga, M., & Harada, E. (2003). Possible regulatory mechanism of DHA-induced anti-stress reaction in rats. *Brain research*, *964*(1), 136-143.

Maes, M., Christophe, A., Bosmans, E., Lin, A., & Neels, H. (2000). In humans, serum polyunsaturated fatty acid levels predict the response of proinflammatory cytokines to psychologic stress. *Biological psychiatry*, *47*(10), 910-920.

Keenan, K., & Hipwell, A. E. (2015). Modulation of prenatal stress via docosahexaenoic acid supplementation: implications for child mental health. *Nutrition reviews*, *73*(3), 166-174.

Hibbeln, J. R. (1998). Fish consumption and major depression. *Lancet*, *351*(9110), 1213.

Hibbeln, J. R. (2002). Seafood consumption, the DHA content of mothers' milk and prevalence rates of postpartum depression: a cross-national, ecological analysis. *Journal of affective disorders*, *69*(1), 15-29.

Golding, J., Steer, C., Emmett, P., Davis, J. M., & Hibbeln, J. R. (2009). High levels of depressive symptoms in pregnancy with low omega-3 fatty acid intake from fish. *Epidemiology*, *20*(4), 598-603.

Strøm, M., Mortensen, E. L., Halldorsson, T. I., Thorsdottir, I., & Olsen, S. F. (2009). Fish and long-chain n− 3 polyunsaturated fatty acid intakes during pregnancy and risk of postpartum depression: a prospective study based on a large national birth cohort. *The American journal of clinical nutrition, 90*(1), 149-155.

Mozurkewich, E. L., Clinton, C. M., Chilimigras, J. L., Hamilton, S. E., Allbaugh, L. J., Berman, D. R., ... & Vahratian, A. M. (2013). The Mothers, Omega-3, and Mental Health Study: a double-blind, randomized controlled trial. *American journal of obstetrics and gynecology, 208*(4), 313-e1.

Freeman, M. P., Hibbeln, J. R., Wisner, K. L., Davis, J. M., Mischoulon, D., Peet, M., ... & Stoll, A. L. (2006). Omega-3 fatty acids: evidence basis for treatment and future research in psychiatry. *Journal of Clinical psychiatry, 67*(12), 1954.

33. How to successfully start a healthy diet change?

Sigman-Grant, M., Warland, R., & Hsieh, G. (2003). Selected lower-fat foods positively impact nutrient quality in diets of free-living Americans. *Journal of the american dietetic association, 103*(5), 570-576.

Stookey, J. D., Constant, F., Gardner, C. D., & Popkin, B. M. (2007). Replacing sweetened caloric beverages with drinking water is associated with lower energy intake. *Obesity, 15*(12), 3013-3022.

Wang, Y. C., Ludwig, D. S., Sonneville, K., & Gortmaker, S. L. (2009). Impact of change in sweetened caloric beverage consumption on energy intake among children and adolescents. *Archives of pediatrics & adolescent medicine, 163*(4), 336-343.

Papathanasopoulos, A., & Camilleri, M. (2010). Dietary fiber supplements: effects in obesity and metabolic syndrome and relationship to gastrointestinal functions. *Gastroenterology*, *138*(1), 65-72.

Verger, E. O., Holmes, B. A., Huneau, J. F., & Mariotti, F. (2014). Simple changes within dietary subgroups can rapidly improve the nutrient adequacy of the diet of French adults. *The Journal of nutrition, 144*(6), 929-936.

Bianchi, C. M., Mariotti, F., Verger, E. O., & Huneau, J. F. (2016). Pregnancy requires major changes in the quality of the diet for nutritional adequacy: simulations in the French and the United States populations. *PloS one, 11*(3), e0149858.

Comerford, K. B., Ayoob, K. T., Murray, R. D., & Atkinson, S. A. (2016). The Role of Avocados in Maternal Diets during the Periconceptional Period, Pregnancy, and Lactation. *Nutrients, 8*(5), 313.

34. What is mindful eating and why is it important?

Framson, C., Kristal, A. R., Schenk, J. M., Littman, A. J., Zeliadt, S., & Benitez, D. (2009). Development and validation of the mindful eating questionnaire. *Journal of the American Dietetic Association, 109*(8), 1439-1444.

Hutchinson, A. D., Charters, M., Prichard, I., Fletcher, C., & Wilson, C. (2017). Understanding maternal dietary choices during pregnancy: The role of social norms and mindful eating. *Appetite, 112*, 227-234.

Wansink, B. (2016). *Slim by design: Mindless eating solutions for everyday life*. Hay House, Inc.

Youngwanichsetha, S., Phumdoung, S., & Ingkathawornwong, T. (2014). The effects of mindfulness eating and yoga exercise on blood sugar levels of pregnant women with gestational diabetes mellitus. *Applied Nursing Research: ANR*, 27(4), 227e230.

Framson, C., Kristal, A. R., Schenk, J. M., Littman, A. J., Zeliadt, S., & Benitez, D. (2009). Development and validation of the mindful eating questionnaire. *Journal of the American Dietetic Association*, 109, 1439e1444.

PART 3: NUTRITION SUPPLEMENTATION

35. What supplements should I take during pregnancy and why?

World Health Organization. (2006). *Standards for Maternal and Neonatal Care. Integrated Management of Pregnancy and Childbirth (IMPAC)*. Geneva: World Health Organization.

World health Organization. (2016). *WHO recommendations on antenatal care for a positive pregnancy experience*. Geneva: World Health Organization.

US Department of Health and Human Services. (2015). *2015–2020 dietary guidelines for Americans*. Washington (DC): USDA.

World Health Organization. (2012). *Guideline: vitamin D supplementation in pregnant women*. World Health Organization.

Vitamin supplementation in pregnancy. *DTB* 2016;**54**:81-84.

36. Introduction to nutrients (1): Folic acid

Antony, A. C. (2007). In utero physiology: role of folic acid in nutrient delivery and fetal development. *The American journal of clinical nutrition*, *85*(2), 598S-603S.

US Preventive Services Task Force. (2009). Folic acid for the prevention of neural tube defects: US Preventive Services Task Force recommendation statement. *Annals of Internal Medicine*, *150*(9), 626.

Wolff, T., Witkop, C. T., Miller, T., & Syed, S. B. (2009). Folic acid supplementation for the prevention of neural tube defects: an update of the evidence for the US Preventive Services Task Force. *Annals of Internal Medicine*, *150*(9), 632-639.

Bibbins-Domingo, K., Grossman, D. C., Curry, S. J., Davidson, K. W., Epling, J. W., García, F. A., ... & Mangione, C. M. (2017). Folic acid supplementation for the prevention of neural tube defects: US Preventive Services Task Force recommendation statement. *Jama*, *317*(2), 183-189.

World Health Organization. (2006). *Iron and Folate Supplementation. Standards for Maternal and Neonatal Care. Integrated Management of Pregnancy and Childbirth (IMPAC)*. Geneva: World Health Organization.

New Zealand Ministry of Health. *Folate/Folic Acid Questions & Answers*. Available online: http:// www.health.govt.nz/our-work/preventative-health-wellness/nutrition/folate-folic-acid (last accessed 2017/8/10)

Lumley, J., Watson, L., Watson, M., & Bower, C. (2001). Periconceptional supplementation with folate and/or multivitamins for preventing neural tube defects. *Cochrane Database Syst Rev*, *3*.

Gao, Y., Sheng, C., Xie, R. H., Sun, W., Asztalos, E., Moddemann, D., ... & Wen, S. W. (2016). New Perspective on

Impact of Folic Acid Supplementation during Pregnancy on Neurodevelopment/Autism in the Offspring Children–A Systematic Review. *PloS one, 11*(11), e0165626.

Steenweg-de Graaff, J., Roza, S. J., Walstra, A. N., El Marroun, H., Steegers, E. A., Jaddoe, V. W., ... & White, T. (2017). Associations of maternal folic acid supplementation and folate concentrations during pregnancy with foetal and child head growth: the Generation R Study. *European journal of nutrition, 56*(1), 65.

Cooke, R. W. I., Lucas, A., Yudkin, P. L. N., & Pryse-Davies, J. (1977). Head circumference as an index of brain weight in the fetus and newborn. *Early human development*, 1(2), 145-149.

Roza, S. J., van Batenburg-Eddes, T., Steegers, E. A., Jaddoe, V. W., Mackenbach, J. P., Hofman, A., ... & Tiemeier, H. (2010). Maternal folic acid supplement use in early pregnancy and child behavioural problems: The Generation R Study. *British journal of nutrition, 103*(3), 445-452.

Roth, C., Magnus, P., Schjølberg, S., Stoltenberg, C., Surén, P., McKeague, I. W., ... & Susser, E. (2011). Folic acid supplements in pregnancy and severe language delay in children. *Jama, 306*(14), 1566-1573.

Surén, P., Roth, C., Bresnahan, M., Haugen, M., Hornig, M., Hirtz, D., ... & Schjølberg, S. (2013). Association between maternal use of folic acid supplements and risk of autism spectrum disorders in children. *Jama, 309*(6), 570-577.

Villamor, E., Rifas-Shiman, S. L., Gillman, M. W., & Oken, E. (2012). Maternal Intake of Methyl-Donor Nutrients and Child

Cognition at 3 Years of Age. *Paediatric and perinatal epidemiology, 26*(4), 328-335.

Julvez, J., Fortuny, J., Mendez, M., Torrent, M., Ribas-Fitó, N., & Sunyer, J. (2009). Maternal use of folic acid supplements during pregnancy and four-year-old neurodevelopment in a population-based birth cohort. *Paediatric and perinatal epidemiology, 23*(3), 199-206.

37. Introduction to nutrients (2): Iron

Alwan, N. A., & Hamamy, H. (2015). Maternal iron status in pregnancy and long-term health outcomes in the offspring. *Journal of pediatric genetics, 4*(02), 111-123.

Benoist, B. D., McLean, E., Egll, I., & Cogswell, M. (2008). *Worldwide prevalence of anaemia 1993-2005: WHO global database on anaemia.*

World Health Organization. (2001). *Iron deficiency anaemia: assessment, prevention and control: a guide for programme managers.*

Bannon, D. I., Portnoy, M. E., Olivi, L., Lees, P. S., Culotta, V. C., & Bressler, J. P. (2002). Uptake of lead and iron by divalent metal transporter 1 in yeast and mammalian cells. *Biochemical and biophysical research communications, 295*(4), 978-984.

Kwong, W. T., Friello, P., & Semba, R. D. (2004). Interactions between iron deficiency and lead poisoning: epidemiology and pathogenesis. *Science of the total environment, 330*(1), 21-37.

Golub, M. S., Hogrefe, C. E., Germann, S. L., Capitanio, J. P., & Lozoff, B. (2006). Behavioral consequences of developmental iron deficiency in infant rhesus monkeys. *Neurotoxicology and teratology*, 28(1), 3-17.

Siddappa, A. M., Georgieff, M. K., Wewerka, S., Worwa, C., Nelson, C. A., & Deregnier, R. A. (2004). Iron deficiency alters auditory recognition memory in newborn infants of diabetic mothers. *Pediatric research*, *55*(6), 1034-1041.

DeBoer, T., Wewerka, S., Bauer, P. J., Georgieff, M. K., & Nelson, C. A. (2005). Explicit memory performance in infants of diabetic mothers at 1 year of age. *Developmental Medicine & Child Neurology*, *47*(8), 525-531.

Riggins, T., Miller, N. C., Bauer, P. J., Georgieff, M. K., & Nelson, C. A. (2009). Consequences of low neonatal iron status due to maternal diabetes mellitus on explicit memory performance in childhood. *Developmental neuropsychology*, *34*(6), 762-779.

Tamura, T., Goldenberg, R. L., Hou, J., Johnston, K. E., Cliver, S. P., Ramey, S. L., & Nelson, K. G. (2002). Cord serum ferritin concentrations and mental and psychomotor development of children at five years of age. *The Journal of pediatrics*, *140*(2), 165-170.

Wachs, T. D., Pollitt, E., Cueto, S., Jacoby, E., & Creed-Kanashiro, H. (2005). Relation of neonatal iron status to individual variability in neonatal temperament. *Developmental psychobiology*, *46*(2), 141-153.

World Health Organization. (2006). *Iron and Folate Supplementation. Standards for Maternal and Neonatal Care. Integrated Management of Pregnancy and Childbirth (IMPAC)*. Geneva: World Health Organization.

Christian, P., Murray-Kolb, L. E., Khatry, S. K., Katz, J., Schaefer, B. A., Cole, P. M., ... & Tielsch, J. M. (2010). Prenatal micronutrient supplementation and intellectual and motor function in early school-aged children in Nepal. *Jama, 304*(24), 2716-2723.

US Department of Health and Human Services. (2015). *2015– 2020 dietary guidelines for Americans*. Washington (DC): USDA.

Ministry of Health New Zealand. 2006 (revised 2008). *Food and Nutrition Guidelines for Healthy Pregnant and Breastfeeding Women: A background paper*. Wellington: Ministry of Health.

38. Introduction to nutrients (3): Vitamin D

World Health Organization. (2012). *Guideline: vitamin D supplementation in pregnant women*. World Health Organization.

Makariou, S., Liberopoulos, E. N., Elisaf, M., & Challa, A. (2011). Novel roles of vitamin D in disease: what is new in 2011?. *European journal of internal medicine, 22*(4), 355-362.

Vitamin supplementation in pregnancy. *DTB* 2016;**54**:81-84.

Hyppönen, E., & Boucher, B. J. (2010). Avoidance of vitamin D deficiency in pregnancy in the United Kingdom: the case for a unified approach in National policy. *British journal of Nutrition, 104*(3), 309-314.

Calvo, M. S., Whiting, S. J., & Barton, C. N. (2005). Vitamin D intake: a global perspective of current status. *The Journal of nutrition, 135*(2), 310-316.

Bodnar, L. M., Catov, J. M., Simhan, H. N., Holick, M. F., Powers, R. W., & Roberts, J. M. (2007). Maternal vitamin D deficiency increases the risk of preeclampsia. *The Journal of Clinical Endocrinology & Metabolism*, *92*(9), 3517-3522.

Zhang, C., Qiu, C., Hu, F. B., David, R. M., Van Dam, R. M., Bralley, A., & Williams, M. A. (2008). Maternal plasma 25-hydroxyvitamin D concentrations and the risk for gestational diabetes mellitus. *PLoS one*, *3*(11), e3753.

Dawodu, A., & Nath, R. (2011). High prevalence of moderately severe vitamin D deficiency in preterm infants. *Pediatrics International*, *53*(2), 207-210.

Leffelaar, E. R., Vrijkotte, T. G., & van Eijsden, M. (2010). Maternal early pregnancy vitamin D status in relation to fetal and neonatal growth: results of the multi-ethnic Amsterdam Born Children and their Development cohort. *British Journal of Nutrition*, *104*(1), 108-117.

Ross, A. C., Taylor, C. L., Yaktine, A. L., & Del Valle, H. B. Food and Nutrition Board. Institute of Medicine. *Dietary Reference Intakes for Calcium and Vitamin D*. 2011.

39. Introduction to nutrients (4): Multiple micronutrient supplements

UNICEF/WHO/UNU. (1999) *Composition of a multi-micronutrient supplement to be used in pilot programmes among pregnant women in developing countries*. UNICEF, NY, USA

McCauley, M. E., van den Broek, N., Dou, L., & Othman, M. (2015). Vitamin A supplementation during pregnancy for maternal and newborn outcomes. *The Cochrane Library*.

Ali, H., Hamadani, J., Mehra, S., Tofail, F., Hasan, M. I., Shaikh, S., ... & Christian, P. (2017). Effect of maternal antenatal and newborn supplementation with vitamin A on cognitive development of school-aged children in rural Bangladesh: a follow-up of a placebo-controlled, randomized trial. *The American Journal of Clinical Nutrition*, ajcn134478.

Zimmermann, M. B. (2009). Iodine deficiency. *Endocrine reviews*, *30*(4), 376-408.

Becker, D. V., Braverman, L. E., Delange, F., Dunn, J. T., Franklyn, J. A., Hollowell, J. G., ... & Rovet, J. F. (2006). Iodine supplementation for pregnancy and lactation—United States and Canada: recommendations of the American Thyroid Association. *Thyroid*, *16*(10), 949-951.

Qian, M., Wang, D., Watkins, W. E., Gebski, V., Yan, Y. Q., & Li, M. (2005). The effects of iodine on intelligence in children: a meta-analysis of studies conducted in China. *Asia Pacific journal of clinical nutrition*, *14*(1), 32.

Haider, B.A., Bhutta, Z.A. (2017). Multiple-micronutrient supplementation for women during pregnancy. *Cochrane Database Syst Rev*. 4:CD004905

Supplementation with Multiple Micronutrients Intervention Trial (SUMMIT) Study Group. (2008). Effect of maternal multiple micronutrient supplementation on fetal loss and infant death in Indonesia: a double-blind cluster-randomised trial. *The Lancet*, *371*(9608), 215-227.

Prado, E. L., Ullman, M. T., Muadz, H., Alcock, K. J., Shankar, A. H., & SUMMIT Study Group. (2012). The effect of maternal multiple micronutrient supplementation on cognition and mood during pregnancy and postpartum in Indonesia: a randomized trial. *PloS one*, *7*(3), e32519.

Prado, E. L., Sebayang, S. K., Apriatni, M., Adawiyah, S. R., Hidayati, N., Islamiyah, A., ... & Ullman, M. T. (2017). Maternal multiple micronutrient supplementation and other biomedical and socioenvironmental influences on children's cognition at age 9–12 years in Indonesia: follow-up of the SUMMIT randomised trial. *The Lancet Global Health*, *5*(2), e217-e228.

40. Introduction to nutrients (5): Omega-3 PUFA

Martinez, M. (1992). Tissue levels of polyunsaturated fatty acids during early human development. *The Journal of pediatrics*, *120*(4), S129-S138.

Lauritzen, L. A., Hansen, H. S., Jørgensen, M. H., & Michaelsen, K. F. (2001). The essentiality of long chain n-3 fatty acids in relation to development and function of the brain and retina. *Progress in lipid research*, *40*(1), 1-94.

Hadders-Algra, M. (2005). The Role of Long-Chain Poly-Unsaturated Fatty Acids (LCPUFA) in Growth and Development. *Early Nutrition and its later consequences: new opportunities*, 80-94.

Bazan, N. G., Molina, M. F., & Gordon, W. C. (2011). Docosahexaenoic acid signalolipidomics in nutrition: significance in aging, neuroinflammation, macular degeneration, Alzheimer's, and other neurodegenerative diseases. *Annual review of nutrition*, *31*, 321-351.

Rogers, L. K., Valentine, C. J., & Keim, S. A. (2013). DHA supplementation: current implications in pregnancy and childhood. *Pharmacological research*, *70*(1), 13-19.

Bertrand, P. C., O'kusky, J. R., & Innis, S. M. (2006). Maternal dietary (n-3) fatty acid deficiency alters neurogenesis in the embryonic rat brain. *The Journal of nutrition*, *136*(6), 1570-1575.

Chmielewska, A., Dziechciarz, P., Gieruszczak-Białek, D., Horvath, A., Pieścik-Lech, M., Ruszczyński, M., ... & Szajewska, H. (2016). Effects of prenatal and/or postnatal supplementation with iron, PUFA or folic acid on neurodevelopment: update. *British Journal of Nutrition*, 1-6.

Dunstan, J. A., Simmer, K., Dixon, G., & Prescott, S. L. (2008). Cognitive assessment of children at age 2½ years after maternal fish oil supplementation in pregnancy: a randomised controlled trial. *Archives of Disease in Childhood-Fetal and Neonatal Edition*, *93*(1), F45-F50.

Helland, I. B., Smith, L., Saarem, K., Saugstad, O. D., & Drevon, C. A. (2003). Maternal supplementation with very-long-chain n-3 fatty acids during pregnancy and lactation augments children's IQ at 4 years of age. *Pediatrics*, *111*(1), e39-e44.

Colombo, J., Gustafson, K. M., Gajewski, B. J., Shaddy, D. J., Kerling, E. H., Thodosoff, J. M., ... & Carlson, S. E. (2016). Prenatal DHA supplementation and infant attention. *Pediatric research*, *80*(5), 656-662.

Mulder, K. A., King, D. J., & Innis, S. M. (2014). Omega-3 fatty acid deficiency in infants before birth identified using a randomized trial of maternal DHA supplementation in pregnancy. *PLoS One*, *9*(1), e83764.

Kannass, K. N., Colombo, J., & Carlson, S. E. (2009). Maternal DHA levels and toddler free-play attention. *Developmental neuropsychology*, *34*(2), 159-174.

Loomans, E. M., Van den Bergh, B. R., Schelling, M., Vrijkotte, T. G., & Van Eijsden, M. (2014). Maternal long-chain polyunsaturated fatty acid status during early pregnancy and children's risk of problem behavior at age 5-6 years. *The Journal of pediatrics*, *164*(4), 762-768.

Campoy, C., Escolano-Margarit, M. V., Ramos, R., Parrilla-Roure, M., Csábi, G., Beyer, J., ... & Koletzko, B. V. (2011). Effects of prenatal fish-oil and 5-methyltetrahydrofolate supplementation on cognitive development of children at 6.5 y of age. *The American journal of clinical nutrition*, *94*(6 Suppl), 1880S-1888S.

Koletzko, B., Cetin, I., & Brenna, J. T. (2007). Dietary fat intakes for pregnant and lactating women. *British Journal of Nutrition*, *98*(5), 873-877.

Koletzko, B., Lien, E., Agostoni, C., Böhles, H., Campoy, C., Cetin, I., ... & Hoesli, I. (2008). The roles of long-chain polyunsaturated fatty acids in pregnancy, lactation and infancy: review of current knowledge and consensus recommendations. *Journal of perinatal medicine*, *36*(1), 5-14.

Patterson, E., Wall, R., Fitzgerald, G. F., Ross, R. P., & Stanton, C. (2012). Health implications of high dietary omega-6 polyunsaturated fatty acids. *Journal of nutrition and metabolism*, *2012*.

41. Introduction to nutrients (6): The ratio of omega-6 to omega-3 PUFA

Souza, R. G., Gomes, A. C., Naves, M. M., & Mota, J. F. (2015). Nuts and legume seeds for cardiovascular risk reduction: scientific evidence and mechanisms of action. *Nutrition reviews*, *73*(6), 335-347.

Kelly, J. H., & Sabaté, J. (2006). Nuts and coronary heart disease: an epidemiological perspective. *British Journal of Nutrition*, *96*(S2), S61-S67.

Jiang, R., Jacobs Jr, D. R., Mayer-Davis, E., Szklo, M., Herrington, D., Jenny, N. S., ... & Barr, R. G. (2005). Nut and seed consumption and inflammatory markers in the multi-ethnic study of atherosclerosis. *American Journal of Epidemiology*, *163*(3), 222-231.

Jiang, R., Manson, J. E., Stampfer, M. J., Liu, S., Willett, W. C., & Hu, F. B. (2002). Nut and peanut butter consumption and risk of type 2 diabetes in women. *Jama*, *288*(20), 2554-2560.

González, C. A., & Salas-Salvadó, J. (2006). The potential of nuts in the prevention of cancer. *British Journal of Nutrition*, *96*(S2), S87-S94.

Steer, C. D., Lattka, E., Koletzko, B., Golding, J., & Hibbeln, J. R. (2013). Maternal fatty acids in pregnancy, FADS polymorphisms, and child intelligence quotient at 8 y of age. *The American journal of clinical nutrition*, *98*(6), 1575-1582.

Harnack, K., Andersen, G., & Somoza, V. (2009). Quantitation of alpha-linolenic acid elongation to eicosapentaenoic and docosahexaenoic acid as affected by the ratio of n6/n3 fatty acids. *Nutrition & metabolism*, *6*(1), 8.

Sakayori, N., Kikkawa, T., Tokuda, H., Kiryu, E., Yoshizaki, K., Kawashima, H., ... & Shibata, H. (2016). Maternal dietary imbalance between omega-6 and omega-3 polyunsaturated fatty acids impairs neocortical development via epoxy metabolites. *Stem Cells*, *34*(2), 470-482.

Kim, H., Kim, H., Lee, E., Kim, Y., Ha, E. H., & Chang, N. (2017). Association between maternal intake of n-6 to n-3 fatty acid ratio during pregnancy and infant neurodevelopment at 6 months of age: results of the MOCEH cohort study. *Nutrition journal*, *16*(1), 23.

Strain, J. J., Davidson, P. W., Bonham, M. P., Duffy, E. M., Stokes-Riner, A., Thurston, S. W., ... & Sloane-Reeves, J. (2008). Associations of maternal long-chain polyunsaturated fatty acids, methyl mercury, and infant development in the Seychelles Child Development Nutrition Study. *Neurotoxicology*, *29*(5), 776-782.

Bernard, J. Y., De Agostini, M., Forhan, A., de Lauzon-Guillain, B., Charles, M. A., Heude, B., & EDEN Mother-Child Cohort Study Group. (2013). The dietary n6: n3 fatty acid ratio during pregnancy is inversely associated with child neurodevelopment in the EDEN mother-child cohort. *The Journal of nutrition*, *143*(9), 1481-1488.

Loomans, E. M., Van den Bergh, B. R., Schelling, M., Vrijkotte, T. G., & Van Eijsden, M. (2014). Maternal long-chain polyunsaturated fatty acid status during early pregnancy and children's risk of problem behavior at age 5-6 years. *The Journal of pediatrics*, *164*(4), 762-768.

Steenweg-de Graaff, J. C., Tiemeier, H., Basten, M. G., Rijlaarsdam, J., Demmelmair, H., Koletzko, B., ... & Roza, S. J. (2014). Maternal LC-PUFA status during pregnancy and child problem behavior: the Generation R Study. *Pediatric research*, *77*(3), 489-497.

Institute of Medicine. (2005). *Dietary reference intakes for energy, carbohydrate, fiber, fat, fatty acids, cholesterol, protein, and amino acids*. Washington D.C.: National Academies Press. pp. 422–588.

Simopoulos, A. P. (2010). The omega-6/omega-3 fatty acid ratio: health implications. *Oléagineux, Corps gras, Lipides*, *17*(5), 267-275.

Simopoulos, A. P. (2011). Evolutionary Aspects of Diet: The Omega-6/Omega-3 Ratio and the Brain. *Molecular Neurobiology*.

Patterson, E., Wall, R., Fitzgerald, G. F., Ross, R. P., & Stanton, C. (2012). Health implications of high dietary omega-6 polyunsaturated fatty acids. *Journal of nutrition and metabolism*, *2012*.

Steenweg-de Graaff, J., Tiemeier, H., Ghassabian, A., Rijlaarsdam, J., Jaddoe, V. W., Verhulst, F. C., & Roza, S. J. (2016). Maternal fatty acid status during pregnancy and child autistic traits: the generation R study. *American journal of epidemiology*, *183*(9), 792-799.

PART 4: FOOD SAFETY & SUBSTANCE ABUSE

42. Can I drink coffee and tea during pregnancy?

American College of Obstetricians and Gynecologists. (2010). ACOG CommitteeOpinion No. 462: Moderate caffeine consumption during pregnancy. *Obstetrics and gynecology*, *116*(2 Pt 1), 467.

Christian, M. S., & Brent, R. L. (2001). Teratogen update: evaluation of the reproductive and developmental risks of caffeine. *Teratology*, *64*(1), 51-78.

Tanaka, H., Nakazawa, K., Arima, M., & Iwasaki, S. (1984). Caffeine and its dimethylxanthines and fetal cerebral development in rat. *Brain and Development*, *6*(4), 355-361.

Anderson, N. L., & Hughes, R. N. (2008). Increased emotional reactivity in rats following exposure to caffeine during adolescence. *Neurotoxicology and teratology*, *30*(3), 195-201.

Soellner, D. E., Grandys, T., & Nuñez, J. L. (2009). Chronic prenatal caffeine exposure impairs novel object recognition and radial arm maze behaviors in adult rats. *Behavioural brain research*, *205*(1), 191-199.

Jacobson, S. W., Fein, G. G., Jacobson, J. L., Schwartz, P. M., & Dowler, J. K. (1984). Neonatal correlates of prenatal exposure to smoking, caffeine, and alcohol. *Infant Behavior and development*, *7*(3), 253-265.

Schmidt, R. J., Romitti, P. A., Burns, T. L., Browne, M. L., Druschel, C. M., & Olney, R. S. (2009). Maternal caffeine consumption and risk of neural tube defects. *Birth Defects*

Research Part A: Clinical and Molecular Teratology, *85*(11), 879-889.

Bekkhus, M., Skjøthaug, T., Nordhagen, R., & Borge, A. I. H. (2010). Intrauterine exposure to caffeine and inattention/overactivity in children. *Acta paediatrica*, *99*(6), 925-928.

Chiu, Y. N., Gau, S. S. F., Tsai, W. C., Soong, W. T., & Shang, C. Y. (2009). Demographic and perinatal factors for behavioral problems among children aged 4–9 in Taiwan. *Psychiatry and clinical neurosciences*, *63*(4), 569-576.

43. Why should I stop eating fried potato chips and cookies?

Becalski, A., Lau, B. P. Y., Lewis, D., & Seaman, S. W. (2003). Acrylamide in foods: Occurrence, sources, and modeling. *Journal of Agricultural and Food Chemistry*, *51*(3), 802-808.

Svensson, K., Abramsson, L., Becker, W., Glynn, A., Hellenäs, K. E., Lind, Y., & Rosen, J. (2003). Dietary intake of acrylamide in Sweden. *Food and Chemical Toxicology*, *41*(11), 1581-1586.

Hagmar, L., Wirfält, E., Paulsson, B., & Törnqvist, M. (2005). Differences in hemoglobin adduct levels of acrylamide in the general population with respect to dietary intake, smoking habits and gender. *Mutation Research/Genetic Toxicology and Environmental Mutagenesis*, *580*(1), 157-165.

Soares, C., Cunha, S., & Fernandes, J. (2006). Determination of acrylamide in coffee and coffee products by GC-MS using an improved SPE clean-up. *Food additives and contaminants*, *23*(12), 1276-1282.

Borda, D., & Alexe, P. (2011). Acrylamide levels in food. *Romanian Journal of Food Science*, *1*(1), 3-15.

Capei, R., Pettini, L., NOSTRO, A. L., & Pesavento, G. (2015). Occurrence of Acrylamide in breakfast cereals and biscuits available in Italy. *Journal of preventive medicine and hygiene*, *56*(4), E190.

Thonning Olesen, P., Olsen, A., Frandsen, H., Frederiksen, K., Overvad, K., & Tjønneland, A. (2008). Acrylamide exposure and incidence of breast cancer among postmenopausal women in the Danish Diet, Cancer and Health Study. *International Journal of Cancer*, *122*(9), 2094-2100.

Hogervorst, J. G., Schouten, L. J., Konings, E. J., Goldbohm, R. A., & van den Brandt, P. A. (2008). Dietary acrylamide intake and the risk of renal cell, bladder, and prostate cancer. *The American journal of clinical nutrition*, *87*(5), 1428-1438.

Naruszewicz, M., Zapolska-Downar, D., Kośmider, A., Nowicka, G., Kozłowska-Wojciechowska, M., Vikström, A. S., & Törnqvist, M. (2009). Chronic intake of potato chips in humans increases the production of reactive oxygen radicals by leukocytes and increases plasma C-reactive protein: a pilot study. *The American journal of clinical nutrition*, *89*(3), 773-777.

El-Sayyad, H. I., El-Gammal, H. L., Habak, L. A., Abdel-Galil, H. M., Fernando, A., Gaur, R. L., & Ouhtit, A. (2011). Structural and ultrastructural evidence of neurotoxic effects of fried potato chips on rat postnatal development. *Nutrition*, *27*(10), 1066-1075.

44. How can soft cheese, raw sprouts, and melons be dangerous?

U.S. Centers for Disease Control and Prevention. *Listeria (Listeriosis)*. https://www.cdc.gov/listeria/index.html (last accessed 2017/07/28)

Bakardjiev, A. I., Theriot, J. A., & Portnoy, D. A. (2006). Listeria monocytogenes traffics from maternal organs to the placenta and back. *PLoS pathogens*, *2*(6), e66.

Janakiraman, V. (2008). Listeriosis in pregnancy: diagnosis, treatment, and prevention. *Reviews in Obstetrics and Gynecology*, *1*(4), 179.

45. How dangerous is smoking to me?

Thielen, A., Klus, H., & Müller, L. (2008). Tobacco smoke: unraveling a controversial subject. *Experimental and Toxicologic Pathology*, *60*(2), 141-156.

US Department of Health and Human Services. (2014). *The health consequences of smoking—50 years of progress: a report of the Surgeon General*. Atlanta, GA: US Department of Health and Human Services, Centers for Disease Control and Prevention, National Center for Chronic Disease Prevention and Health Promotion, Office on Smoking and Health, 17.

Hayashi, K., Matsuda, Y., Kawamichi, Y., Shiozaki, A., & Saito, S. (2011). Smoking during pregnancy increases risks of various obstetric complications: a case-cohort study of the Japan Perinatal Registry Network database. *Journal of epidemiology*, *21*(1), 61-66.

Leonardi-Bee, J., Britton, J., & Venn, A. (2011). Secondhand smoke and adverse fetal outcomes in nonsmoking pregnant women: a meta-analysis. *Pediatrics*, *127*(4), 734-741.

46. Does smoking affect my baby?

Lambers, D. S., & Clark, K. E. (1996, April). The maternal and fetal physiologic effects of nicotine. In *Seminars in perinatology* (Vol. 20, No. 2, pp. 115-126). WB Saunders.

Slotkin, T. A. (1998). Fetal nicotine or cocaine exposure: which one is worse?. *Journal of pharmacology and experimental therapeutics*, *285*(3), 931-945.

US Department of Health and Human Services. (2014). *The health consequences of smoking—50 years of progress: a report of the Surgeon General*. Atlanta, GA: US Department of Health and Human Services, Centers for Disease Control and Prevention, National Center for Chronic Disease Prevention and Health Promotion, Office on Smoking and Health, 17.

Mund, M., Louwen, F., Klingelhoefer, D., & Gerber, A. (2013). Smoking and pregnancy—a review on the first major environmental risk factor of the unborn. *International journal of environmental research and public health*, *10*(12), 6485-6499.

Mathews, F., Yudkin, P., Smith, R. F., & Neil, A. (2000). Nutrient intakes during pregnancy: the influence of smoking status and age. *Journal of Epidemiology & Community Health*, *54*(1), 17-23.

Malik, S., Cleves, M. A., Honein, M. A., Romitti, P. A., Botto, L. D., Yang, S., & Hobbs, C. A. (2008). Maternal smoking and congenital heart defects. *Pediatrics*, *121*(4), e810-e816.

Hackshaw, A., Rodeck, C., & Boniface, S. (2011). Maternal smoking in pregnancy and birth defects: a systematic review based on 173 687 malformed cases and 11.7 million controls. *Human reproduction update*, *17*(5), 589-604.

Bublitz, M. H., & Stroud, L. R. (2011). Maternal smoking during pregnancy and offspring brain structure and function: review and agenda for future research. *Nicotine & tobacco research, 14*(4), 388-397.

Polanska, K., Jurewicz, J., & Hanke, W. (2015). Smoking and alcohol drinking during pregnancy as the risk factors for poor child neurodevelopment–A review of epidemiological studies. *International journal of occupational medicine and environmental health.*

Liu, T., Gatsonis, C. A., Baylin, A., Kubzansky, L. D., Loucks, E. B., & Buka, S. L. (2011). Maternal smoking during pregnancy and anger temperament among adult offspring. *Journal of psychiatric research, 45*(12), 1648-1654.

Langley, K., Heron, J., Smith, G. D., & Thapar, A. (2012). Maternal and paternal smoking during pregnancy and risk of ADHD symptoms in offspring: testing for intrauterine effects. *American journal of epidemiology, 176*(3), 261-268.

Riedel, C., Schönberger, K., Yang, S., Koshy, G., Chen, Y. C., Gopinath, B., ... & von Kries, R. (2014). Parental smoking and childhood obesity: higher effect estimates for maternal smoking in pregnancy compared with paternal smoking—a meta-analysis. *International journal of epidemiology, 43*(5), 1593-1606.

47. Should family members stop smoking during pregnancy?

Riedel, C., Schönberger, K., Yang, S., Koshy, G., Chen, Y. C., Gopinath, B., ... & von Kries, R. (2014). Parental smoking and childhood obesity: higher effect estimates for maternal smoking in pregnancy compared with paternal smoking—a meta-analysis. *International journal of epidemiology*, *43*(5), 1593-1606.

Langley, K., Heron, J., Smith, G. D., & Thapar, A. (2012). Maternal and paternal smoking during pregnancy and risk of ADHD symptoms in offspring: testing for intrauterine effects. *American journal of epidemiology*, *176*(3), 261-268.

Flemming, K., Graham, H., McCaughan, D., Angus, K., & Bauld, L. (2015). The barriers and facilitators to smoking cessation experienced by women's partners during pregnancy and the post-partum period: a systematic review of qualitative research. *BMC public health*, *15*(1), 849.

48. Why should I avoid any alcohol?

Riley, E. P., Infante, M. A., & Warren, K. R. (2011). Fetal alcohol spectrum disorders: an overview. *Neuropsychology review*, *21*(2), 73.

Mattson, S. N., Crocker, N., & Nguyen, T. T. (2011). Fetal alcohol spectrum disorders: neuropsychological and behavioral features. *Neuropsychology review*, *21*(2), 81-101.

Weiss, L. A., & Chambers, C. D. (2013). Associations between multivitamin supplement use and alcohol consumption before pregnancy: Pregnancy risk assessment monitoring system, 2004 to 2008. *Alcoholism: Clinical and Experimental Research*, *37*(9), 1595-1600.

Keen, C. L., Uriu-Adams, J. Y., Skalny, A., Grabeklis, A., Grabeklis, S., Green, K., ... & Chambers, C. D. (2010). The plausibility of maternal nutritional status being a contributing factor to the risk for fetal alcohol spectrum disorders: the potential influence of zinc status as an example. *Biofactors, 36*(2), 125-135.

Polanska, K., Jurewicz, J., & Hanke, W. (2015). Smoking and alcohol drinking during pregnancy as the risk factors for poor child neurodevelopment–A review of epidemiological studies. *International journal of occupational medicine and environmental health.*

Sayal, K., Heron, J., Golding, J., & Emond, A. (2007). Prenatal alcohol exposure and gender differences in childhood mental health problems: a longitudinal population-based study. *Pediatrics, 119*(2), e426-e434.

49. Toxic chemicals (1): Cocaine

Mayes, L. C. (1999). Developing brain and in utero cocaine exposure: effects on neural ontogeny. *Development and psychopathology, 11*(4), 685-714.

Dennis, T., Bendersky, M., Ramsay, D., & Lewis, M. (2006). Reactivity and regulation in children prenatally exposed to cocaine. *Developmental psychology, 42*(4), 688.

Linares, T. J., Singer, L. T., Kirchner, H. L., Short, E. J., Min, M. O., Hussey, P., & Minnes, S. (2005). Mental health outcomes of cocaine-exposed children at 6 years of age. *Journal of Pediatric Psychology, 31*(1), 85-97.

Avants, B. B., Hurt, H., Giannetta, J. M., Epstein, C. L., Shera, D. M., Rao, H., ... & Gee, J. C. (2007). Effects of heavy in utero cocaine exposure on adolescent caudate morphology. *Pediatric neurology, 37*(4), 275-279.

Liu, J., Lester, B. M., Neyzi, N., Sheinkopf, S. J., Gracia, L., Kekatpure, M., & Kosofsky, B. E. (2013). Regional brain morphometry and impulsivity in adolescents following prenatal exposure to cocaine and tobacco. *JAMA pediatrics*, *167*(4), 348-354.

Rando, K., Chaplin, T. M., Potenza, M. N., Mayes, L., & Sinha, R. (2013). Prenatal cocaine exposure and gray matter volume in adolescent boys and girls: relationship to substance use initiation. *Biological psychiatry*, *74*(7), 482-489.

50. Toxic chemicals (2): Cannabis

Ashton, C. H. (2001). Pharmacology and effects of cannabis: a brief review. *The British Journal of Psychiatry*, *178*(2), 101-106.

Gunn, J. K. L., Rosales, C. B., Center, K. E., Nuñez, A., Gibson, S. J., Christ, C., & Ehiri, J. E. (2016). Prenatal exposure to cannabis and maternal and child health outcomes: a systematic review and meta-analysis. *BMJ open*, *6*(4), e009986.

El Marroun, H., Tiemeier, H., Steegers, E. A., Jaddoe, V. W., Hofman, A., Verhulst, F. C., ... & Huizink, A. C. (2009). Intrauterine cannabis exposure affects fetal growth trajectories: the Generation R Study. *Journal of the American Academy of Child & Adolescent Psychiatry*, *48*(12), 1173-1181.

Goldschmidt, L., Day, N. L., & Richardson, G. A. (2000). Effects of prenatal marijuana exposure on child behavior problems at age 10. *Neurotoxicology and teratology*, *22*(3), 325-336.

Fried, P. A., Watkinson, B., & Gray, R. (1992). A follow-up study of attentional behavior in 6-year-old children exposed prenatally to marihuana, cigarettes, and alcohol. *Neurotoxicology and teratology*, *14*(5), 299-311.

51. Toxic chemicals (3): Methamphetamine

Kuczkowski, K. M. (2007). The effects of drug abuse on pregnancy. *Current Opinion in Obstetrics and Gynecology*, *19*(6), 578-585.

Plessinger, M. A. (1998). Prenatal exposure to amphetamines: risks and adverse outcomes in pregnancy. *Obstetrics and gynecology clinics of North America*, *25*(1), 119-138.

Smith, L. M., Diaz, S., LaGasse, L. L., Wouldes, T., Derauf, C., Newman, E., ... & Della Grotta, S. (2015). Developmental and behavioral consequences of prenatal methamphetamine exposure: a review of the infant development, environment, and lifestyle (IDEAL) study. *Neurotoxicology and teratology*, *51*, 35-44.

Shah, R., Diaz, S. D., Arria, A., LaGasse, L. L., Derauf, C., Newman, E., ... & Della Grotta, S. (2012). Prenatal methamphetamine exposure and short-term maternal and infant medical outcomes. *American journal of perinatology*, *29*(05), 391-400.

Billing, L., Eriksson, M., Steneroth, G., & Zetterström, R. (1988). Predictive indicators for adjustment in 4-year-old children whose mothers used amphetamine during pregnancy. *Child abuse & neglect*, *12*(4), 503-507.

Twomey, J., LaGasse, L., Derauf, C., Newman, E., Shah, R., Smith, L., ... & Dansereau, L. (2013). Prenatal methamphetamine exposure, home environment, and primary caregiver risk factors predict child behavioral problems at 5 years. *American Journal of Orthopsychiatry, 83*(1), 64-72.

Billing, L., Eriksson, M., Jonsson, B., Steneroth, G., & Zetterstrom, R. (1994). The influence of environmental factors on behavioural problems in 8-year-old children exposed to amphetamine during fetal life. *Child Abuse and Neglect*, 18, 3–9.

Cernerud, L. A. R. S., Eriksson, M., Jonsson, B., Steneroth, G., & Zetterstrom, R. (1996). Amphetamine addiction during pregnancy: 14-year follow-up of growth and school performance. *Acta paediatrica, 85*(2), 204-208.

Chang, L., Smith, L. M., LoPresti, C., Yonekura, M. L., Kuo, J., Walot, I., & Ernst, T. (2004). Smaller subcortical volumes and cognitive deficits in children with prenatal methamphetamine exposure. *Psychiatry Research: Neuroimaging, 132*(2), 95-106.

PART 5: WORK, PHYSICAL EXERCISE, & ENVIRONMENTAL RISKS

52. Does my job affect my baby?

Hobel, C., & Culhane, J. (2003). Role of psychosocial and nutritional stress on poor pregnancy outcome. *The Journal of nutrition, 133*(5), 1709S-1717S.

Bonzini, M., Coggon, D., & Palmer, K. T. (2006). Risk of prematurity, low birth weight, and pre-eclampsia in relation to working hours and physical activities: a systematic review. *Occupational and environmental medicine.*

van Beukering, M. D. M., van Melick, M. J. G. J., Mol, B. W., Frings-Dresen, M. H. W., & Hulshof, C. T. J. (2014). Physically demanding work and preterm delivery: a systematic review and meta-analysis. *International archives of occupational and environmental health*, *87*(8), 809-834.

53. Why I should live and work in a quiet, non-noisy place?

Berglund, B., Lindvall, T., & Schwela, D. H. (1999). Guidelines for community noise. In *Guidelines for community noise*. OMS.

Basner, M., Babisch, W., Davis, A., Brink, M., Clark, C., Janssen, S., & Stansfeld, S. (2014). Auditory and non-auditory effects of noise on health. *The Lancet*, *383*(9925), 1325-1332.

Rehm, S., & Jansen, G. (1978). Aircraft noise and premature birth. *Journal of Sound and Vibration*, *59*(1), 133-135.

Ristovska, G., Laszlo, H. E., & Hansell, A. L. (2014). Reproductive outcomes associated with noise exposure—a systematic review of the literature. *International journal of environmental research and public health*, *11*(8), 7931-7952.

Kim, C. H., Lee, S. C., Shin, J. W., Chung, K. J., Lee, S. H., Shin, M. S., ... & Kim, K. H. (2013). Exposure to music and noise during pregnancy influences neurogenesis and thickness in motor and somatosensory cortex of rat pups. *International neurourology journal*, *17*(3), 107.

54. Should I stop shiftwork during pregnancy?

Costa, G. (2010). Shift work and health: current problems and preventive actions. *Safety and health at Work*, *1*(2), 112-123.

Mozurkewich, E. L., Luke, B., Avni, M., & Wolf, F. M. (2000). Working conditions and adverse pregnancy outcome: a meta-analysis. *Obstetrics & Gynecology*, *95*(4), 623-635.

Bonzini, M., Coggon, D., & Palmer, K. T. (2006). Risk of prematurity, low birth weight, and pre-eclampsia in relation to working hours and physical activities: a systematic review. *Occupational and environmental medicine.*

Bonzini, M., Palmer, K. T., Coggon, D., Carugno, M., Cromi, A., & Ferrario, M. M. (2011). Shift work and pregnancy outcomes: a systematic review with meta-analysis of currently available epidemiological studies. *BJOG: An International Journal of Obstetrics & Gynaecology, 118*(12), 1429-1437.

Roman, E., & Karlsson, O. (2013). Increased anxiety-like behavior but no cognitive impairments in adult rats exposed to constant light conditions during perinatal development. *Upsala journal of medical sciences, 118*(4), 222-227.

Radhakrishnan, A., Aswathy, B. S., Kumar, V. M., & Gulia, K. K. (2015). Sleep deprivation during late pregnancy produces hyperactivity and increased risk-taking behavior in offspring. *Brain research, 1596,* 88-98.

Gulia, K. K., Patel, N., Radhakrishnan, A., & Kumar, V. M. (2014). Reduction in ultrasonic vocalizations in pups born to rapid eye movement sleep restricted mothers in rat model. *PloS one, 9*(1), e84948.

Fujioka, A., Fujioka, T., Tsuruta, R., Izumi, T., Kasaoka, S., & Maekawa, T. (2011). Effects of a constant light environment on hippocampal neurogenesis and memory in mice. *Neuroscience letters, 488*(1), 41-44.

Peng, Y., Wang, W., Tan, T., He, W., Dong, Z., Wang, Y. T., & Han, H. (2016). Maternal sleep deprivation at different stages of pregnancy impairs the emotional and cognitive functions, and suppresses hippocampal long-term potentiation in the offspring rats. *Molecular brain*, 9(1), 17.

Smarr, B. L., Grant, A. D., Perez, L., Zucker, I., & Kriegsfeld, L. J. (2017). Maternal and Early-Life Circadian Disruption Have Long-Lasting Negative Consequences on Offspring Development and Adult Behavior in Mice. *Scientific Reports*, 7.

55. Is physical exercise recommended during pregnancy?

Chen, C. (2017). *Psychology for Pregnancy: How Your Mental Health During Pregnancy Programs Your Baby's Developing Brain*. London: Brain & Life Publishing

Molteni, R., Wu, A., Vaynman, S., Ying, Z., Barnard, R. J., & Gomez-Pinilla, F. (2004). Exercise reverses the harmful effects of consumption of a high-fat diet on synaptic and behavioral plasticity associated to the action of brain-derived neurotrophic factor. *Neuroscience*, 123(2), 429-440.

Hawkins, M., Braun, B., Marcus, B. H., Stanek, E., Markenson, G., & Chasan-Taber, L. (2015). The impact of an exercise intervention on C-reactive protein during pregnancy: a randomized controlled trial. *BMC pregnancy and childbirth*, 15(1), 139.

Jukic, A. M. Z., Lawlor, D. A., Juhl, M., Owe, K. M., Lewis, B., Liu, J., ... & Longnecker, M. P. (2013). Physical activity during pregnancy and language development in the offspring. *Paediatric and perinatal epidemiology*, 27(3), 283-293.

Polańska, K., Muszyński, P., Sobala, W., Dziewirska, E., Merecz-Kot, D., & Hanke, W. (2015). Maternal lifestyle during pregnancy and child psychomotor development—Polish Mother and Child Cohort study. *Early human development*, 91(5), 317-325.

56. What are the benefits of utilizing green environments?

van den Berg, M., Wendel-Vos, W., van Poppel, M., Kemper, H., van Mechelen, W., & Maas, J. (2015). Health benefits of green spaces in the living environment: A systematic review of epidemiological studies. *Urban Forestry & Urban Greening*, *14*(4), 806-816.

Velarde, M. D., Fry, G., & Tveit, M. (2007). Health effects of viewing landscapes–Landscape types in environmental psychology. *Urban Forestry & Urban Greening*, 6(4), 199-212.

World Health Organization. (2016). *Urban Green Spaces and Health–A Review of Evidence*. Geneva, Switzerland: WHO.

Alcock, I., White, M. P., Wheeler, B. W., Fleming, L. E., & Depledge, M. H. (2014). Longitudinal effects on mental health of moving to greener and less green urban areas. *Environmental science & technology*, *48*(2), 1247-1255.

Kaplan, R. (2001). The nature of the view from home: Psychological benefits. *Environment and behavior*, *33*(4), 507-542.

Dzhambov, A. M., Dimitrova, D. D., & Dimitrakova, E. D. (2014). Association between residential greenness and birth weight: Systematic review and meta-analysis. *Urban forestry & urban greening*, *13*(4), 621-629.

Grazuleviciene, R., Danileviciute, A., Dedele, A., Vencloviene, J., Andrusaityte, S., Uždanaviciute, I., & Nieuwenhuijsen, M. J.

(2015). Surrounding greenness, proximity to city parks and pregnancy outcomes in Kaunas cohort study. *International journal of hygiene and environmental health, 218*(3), 358-365.

57. Does air pollution affect me?

Baillie-Hamilton, P. F. (2002). Chemical toxins: a hypothesis to explain the global obesity epidemic. *The Journal of Alternative & Complementary Medicine, 8*(2), 185-192.

Riedl, M. A. (2008). The effect of air pollution on asthma and allergy. *Current allergy and asthma reports, 8*(2), 139-146.

Brook, R. D., Rajagopalan, S., Pope, C. A., Brook, J. R., Bhatnagar, A., Diez-Roux, A. V., ... & Peters, A. (2010). Particulate matter air pollution and cardiovascular disease. *Circulation, 121*(21), 2331-2378.

Block, M. L., & Calderón-Garcidueñas, L. (2009). Air pollution: mechanisms of neuroinflammation and CNS disease. *Trends in neurosciences, 32*(9), 506-516.

58. Does air pollution affect my baby?

de Melo, J. O., Soto, S. F., Katayama, I. A., Wenceslau, C. F., Pires, A. G., Veras, M. M., ... & Heimann, J. C. (2015). Inhalation of fine particulate matter during pregnancy increased IL-4 cytokine levels in the fetal portion of the placenta. *Toxicology letters, 232*(2), 475-480.

Sun, X., Luo, X., Zhao, C., Zhang, B., Tao, J., Yang, Z., ... & Liu, T. (2016). The associations between birth weight and exposure to fine particulate matter (PM 2.5) and its chemical constituents during pregnancy: A meta-analysis. *Environmental Pollution*, *211*, 38-47.

Michikawa, T., Morokuma, S., Fukushima, K., Kato, K., Nitta, H., & Yamazaki, S. (2017). Maternal exposure to air pollutants during the first trimester and foetal growth in Japanese term infants. *Environmental Pollution*, *230*, 387-393.

Vafeiadi, M., Georgiou, V., Chalkiadaki, G., Rantakokko, P., Kiviranta, H., Karachaliou, M., ... & Kyrtopoulos, S. A. (2015). Association of prenatal exposure to persistent organic pollutants with obesity and cardiometabolic traits in early childhood: the Rhea mother–child cohort (Crete, Greece). *Environmental health perspectives*, *123*(10), 1015.

Rundle, A., Hoepner, L., Hassoun, A., Oberfield, S., Freyer, G., Holmes, D., ... & Whyatt, R. (2012). Association of childhood obesity with maternal exposure to ambient air polycyclic aromatic hydrocarbons during pregnancy. *American journal of epidemiology*, *175*(11), 1163-1172.

Guxens, M., Aguilera, I., Ballester, F., Estarlich, M., Fernández-Somoano, A., Lertxundi, A., ... & Sunyer, J. (2012). Prenatal exposure to residential air pollution and infant mental development: modulation by antioxidants and detoxification factors. *Environmental health perspectives*, *120*(1), 144.

World Health Organization. (2016). *WHO global urban ambient air pollution database (update 2016)*. Geneva. Diunduh.

59. Toxic chemicals (4): Lead

U.S. Center for Disease Control and Prevention. *Sources of Lead.* https://www.cdc.gov/nceh/lead/tips/sources.htm (last accessed 2017/07/27)

U.S. Center for Disease Control and Prevention. *Lead Prevention Tips.* https://www.cdc.gov/nceh/lead/tips.htm (last accessed 2017/07/27)

Needleman, H. (2004). Lead poisoning. *Annu. Rev. Med.*, *55*, 209-222.

Jedrychowski, W., Perera, F. P., Jankowski, J., Mrozek-Budzyn, D., Mroz, E., Flak, E., ... & Lisowska-Miszczyk, I. (2009). Very low prenatal exposure to lead and mental development of children in infancy and early childhood. *Neuroepidemiology*, *32*(4), 270-278.

Vigeh, M., Yokoyama, K., Matsukawa, T., Shinohara, A., & Ohtani, K. (2014). Low level prenatal blood lead adversely affects early childhood mental development. *Journal of child neurology*, *29*(10), 1305-1311.

Wasserman, G. A., Liu, X., Popovac, D., Factor-Litvak, P., Kline, J., Waternaux, C., ... & Graziano, J. H. (2000). The Yugoslavia Prospective Lead Study: contributions of prenatal and postnatal lead exposure to early intelligence. *Neurotoxicology and Teratology*, *22*(6), 811-818.

Ashley Alvarado (2010) Why should I be concerned about lead in jewelry? http://californiawatch.org/react-and-act/why-should-i-be-concerned-about-lead-jewelry (last accessed 2017/07/27)

Shah-Kulkarni, S., Ha, M., Kim, B. M., Kim, E., Hong, Y. C., Park, H., ... & Kim, Y. J. (2016). Neurodevelopment in early childhood affected by prenatal lead exposure and iron intake. *Medicine*, 95(4).

PART 6: SLEEP

60. What are the typical sleep problems during pregnancy?

Brunner, D. P., Münch, M., Biedermann, K., Huch, R., Huch, A., & Borbély, A. A. (1994). Changes in sleep and sleep electroencephalogram during pregnancy. *Sleep*, *17*(7), 576-582.

Lee, K. A. (1998). Alterations in sleep during pregnancy and postpartum: a review of 30 years of research. *Sleep medicine reviews*, *2*(4), 231-242.

Lee, K. A., Zaffke, M. E., & McEnany, G. (2000). Parity and sleep patterns during and after pregnancy. *Obstetrics & Gynecology*, *95*(1), 14-18.

Hanif, S. (2006). Frequency and pattern of urinary complaints among pregnant women. *Journal of the College of Physicians and Surgeons--Pakistan: JCPSP*, *16*(8), 514-517.

Okun, M. L., & Coussons-Read, M. E. (2007). Sleep disruption during pregnancy: how does it influence serum cytokines?. *Journal of reproductive immunology*, *73*(2), 158-165.

Chang, J. J., Pien, G. W., Duntley, S. P., & Macones, G. A. (2010). Sleep deprivation during pregnancy and maternal and fetal outcomes: is there a relationship?. *Sleep medicine reviews*, *14*(2), 107-114.

Mindell, J. A., Cook, R. A., & Nikolovski, J. (2015). Sleep patterns and sleep disturbances across pregnancy. *Sleep medicine*, *16*(4), 483-488.

61. How much sleep is necessary?

Hirshkowitz, M., Whiton, K., Albert, S. M., Alessi, C., Bruni, O., DonCarlos, L., ... & Neubauer, D. N. (2015). National Sleep Foundation's sleep time duration recommendations: methodology and results summary. *Sleep Health*, *1*(1), 40-43.

Chen, C. (2017). *Plato's Insight: How Physical Exercise Boosts Mental Excellence.* London: Brain & Life Publishing

62. How does insufficient and poor sleep affect me?

Chen, C. (2017). *Plato's Insight: How Physical Exercise Boosts Mental Excellence.* London: Brain & Life Publishing

Jomeen, J., & Martin, C. R. (2007). Assessment and relationship of sleep quality to depression in early pregnancy. *Journal of Reproductive and Infant Psychology*, *25*(1), 87-99.

Ross, L. E., Murray, B. J., & Steiner, M. (2005). Sleep and perinatal mood disorders: a critical review. *Journal of Psychiatry and Neuroscience*, *30*(4), 247.

Okun, M. L. (2015). Sleep and postpartum depression. *Current opinion in psychiatry*, *28*(6), 490-496.

O'Keeffe, M., & St-Onge, M. P. (2013). Sleep duration and disorders in pregnancy: implications for glucose metabolism and pregnancy outcomes. *International Journal of Obesity*, *37*(6), 765-770.

Facco, F. L., Grobman, W. A., Kramer, J., Ho, K. H., & Zee, P. C. (2010). Self-reported short sleep duration and frequent snoring in pregnancy: impact on glucose metabolism. *American journal of obstetrics and gynecology*, *203*(2), 142-e1.

Palagini, L., Gemignani, A., Banti, S., Manconi, M., Mauri, M., & Riemann, D. (2014). Chronic sleep loss during pregnancy as a determinant of stress: impact on pregnancy outcome. *Sleep medicine*, *15*(8), 853-859.

Lee, K. A., & Gay, C. L. (2004). Sleep in late pregnancy predicts length of labor and type of delivery. *American journal of obstetrics and gynecology*, *191*(6), 2041-2046.

63. Does my sleep affect my baby?

Chang, J. J., Pien, G. W., Duntley, S. P., & Macones, G. A. (2010). Sleep deprivation during pregnancy and maternal and fetal outcomes: is there a relationship?. *Sleep medicine reviews*, *14*(2), 107-114.

Okun, M. L., Schetter, C. D., & Glynn, L. M. (2011). Poor sleep quality is associated with preterm birth. *Sleep*, *34*(11), 1493-1498.

Palagini, L., Gemignani, A., Banti, S., Manconi, M., Mauri, M., & Riemann, D. (2014). Chronic sleep loss during pregnancy as a determinant of stress: impact on pregnancy outcome. *Sleep medicine*, *15*(8), 853-859.

Samaraweera, Y., & Abeysena, C. (2010). Maternal sleep deprivation, sedentary lifestyle and cooking smoke: Risk factors for miscarriage: A case control study. *Australian and New Zealand Journal of Obstetrics and Gynaecology*, *50*(4), 352-357.

Abeysena, C., Jayawardana, P., & Seneviratne, R. D. A. (2010). Effect of psychosocial stress and physical activity on low birthweight: a cohort study. *Journal of Obstetrics and Gynaecology Research*, *36*(2), 296-303.

64. What if I snore?

Micheli, K., Komninos, I., Bagkeris, E., Roumeliotaki, T., Koutis, A., Kogevinas, M., & Bourjeily, G., Raker, C. A., Chalhoub, M., & Miller, M. A. (2010). Sleep disordered breathing symptoms in pregnancy and adverse pregnancy and fetal outcomes. *European Respiratory Journal*, erj00218-2010.

Chatzi, L. (2011). Sleep patterns in late pregnancy and risk of preterm birth and fetal growth restriction. *Epidemiology*, *22*(5), 738-744.

66. How can I improve sleep quality?

Chen, C. (2017). *Plato's Insight: How Physical Exercise Boosts Mental Excellence.* London: Brain & Life Publishing

Takahashi, M. (2003). The role of prescribed napping in sleep medicine. *Sleep medicine reviews*, *7*(3), 227-235.

Lovato, N., & Lack, L. (2010). 9 The effects of napping on cognitive functioning. *Progress in brain research*, *185*, 155.

National Sleep Foundation. *Healthy sleep tips*. Available https://sleepfoundation.org/sleep-tools-tips/healthy-sleep-tips (last accessed 2017/07/26)

INDEX

acrylamide, 86, 88, 92

ADHD, 35, 42, 50, 51, 55, 57, 83, 96, 97, 99, 101

aggressive, 35, 50, 96, 102

alcohol, 10, 13, 14, 33, 98, 100, 127

anemia, 18, 19, 66, 68, 70, 71, 76

anxiety, 26, 35, 51, 59, 60, 69, 83, 101, 108, 109, 112, 122

autism, 51, 69, 83

BDNF, 6, 7, 34, 54, 110, 122, 123

BMI, 24, 52, 56

breastfeed, 19, 55

butter, 32, 33, 40, 46, 48

caffeine, 10, 86, 87, 127

calcium, 47, 48, 73

cancer, 27, 36, 47, 49, 73, 82, 88, 92, 108

cardiovascular disease, 24, 36, 42, 49, 52, 82, 92, 106, 108, 114, 126

cereal, 32, 33, 72, 88

cerebellum, 86, 95

cesarean, 53, 57, 59, 122

cheese, 48, 89

chemical, 5, 49, 59, 88, 92, 94, 99, 100, 101, 104, 117, 127

coffee, 11, 86, 87, 88

cognitive, 4, 7, 24, 25, 27, 36, 37, 38, 42, 51, 52, 77, 78, 79, 83, 95, 96, 98, 99, 102, 106, 111, 112, 122, 126

communication, 7, 42, 83

cortex, 86, 95, 99, 107

cortisol, 6, 7, 26, 34, 51, 52, 54, 108, 111, 122, 123

dairy, 28, 33, 35, 47, 48, 73, 76, 77, 89

delivery, 11, 17, 20, 26, 37, 57, 59, 71, 93, 120

depression, 7, 35, 51, 53, 60, 69, 83, 87, 96, 101, 108, 110, 112, 122, 126

DHA, 17, 29, 60, 79, 80, 81

diabete, 24, 27, 34, 47, 49, 51, 52, 59, 63, 73, 82, 92, 108, 112, 122

education, 2, 77, 78, 207

emotional, 1, 52, 55, 62, 67, 70, 80, 83, 96, 99, 102, 122

energy intake, 10, 30, 31, 58

EPA, 29, 60, 79, 80, 81

executive function, 22, 23, 26, 99, 101

first trimester, 18, 19, 22, 30, 56, 98, 105, 120

fish, 32, 33, 34, 40, 42, 43, 45, 46, 60, 73, 81, 82, 83

folic acid, 13, 19, 66, 68, 69, 71

fruit, 10, 11, 15, 28, 31, 32, 33, 34, 36, 37, 38, 61, 72, 116

growth restriction, 7, 24, 124

head, 23, 68, 69, 100, 101, 106

high-fat, 15, 51, 58, 61

hypertension, 7, 34, 47, 53, 59, 93, 101, 106

infection, 7, 24, 27, 53, 76, 89, 90

inflammation, 6, 7, 34, 51, 82, 88, 110, 114, 115

intelligence, 5, 6, 8, 22, 26, 99, 101, 110, 129

iodine, 47, 76

IQ, 42, 45, 71, 77, 78, 80, 82, 95, 101, → intelligence

iron, 19, 29, 41, 58, 66, 67, 70, 71, 72, 77, 118, 190

juice, 32, 36, 38, 39, 61, 72, 91

junk food, 36, 51, 62

language, 24, 69, 71, 78, 80, 83, 102, 110

legume, 33, 39, 40, 72

low birth weight, 7, 12, 19, 24, 54, 67, 77, 78, 100, 108, 113, 115, 123, 124

macrosomia, 57, 59

meat, 32, 33, 40, 49, 61, 72, 77, 90, 91, 118

Mediterranean, 33, 34, 35, 58, 116

mercury, 43, 45, 46

micronutrient, 6, 14, 54, 66, 67, 70, 75, 76

milk, 31, 32, 37, 48, 61, 73, 89, 90

mindful, 58, 62, 63

miscarriage, 54, 89, 108, 123

monounsaturated fatty acid, 34, 47, 79

mortality, 20, 67, 78

motor, 42, 43, 69, 71, 78, 83, 102, 107

multiple micronutrient supplement, 14, 67, 75

neonatal intensive care, 54, 100, 101

neural tube defect, 13, 54, 66, 68, 87

neurogenesis, 4, 7, 82, 107, 109

neuron, 4, 6, 7, 13, 79, 82, 86, 88, 95, 98, 99, 107, 110

obesity, 22, 26, 34, 49, 50, 51, 52, 54, 55, 57, 58, 62, 96, 97, 114, 115, 116, 121

omega-3, 17, 29, 34, 41, 42, 43, 60, 79, 82, 83

overweight, 26, 52, 55, 57, 58, 96, 97

pain, 96, 117, 118, 120

physical exercise, 5, 10, 11, 58, 110, 111

placental, 7, 51, 54, 89, 93, 94

potato chips, 61, 88

poultry, 33, 40

pre-eclampsia, 52, 73, 108

preterm birth, 7, 24, 28, 34, 54, 57, 67, 73, 89, 104, 105, 106, 108, 113, 123, 124

pro-inflammatory, 6, 52, 54, 60, 108, 114, 122, 123, → inflammation

protein, 26, 34, 40, 41, 47, 117

seafood, 40, 41, 42, 43, 45, 46, 60, 72, 77, 81, 83, 91, → fish

second trimester, 19, 30, 80, 120, 123

single mother, 15

sleep, 2, 5, 106, 108, 120, 121, 122, 123, 124, 125, 126, 127, 128

smoking, 10, 11, 13, 15, 49, 92, 94, 95, 97

snack, 28, 31, 32, 49, 61, 62, 88, 127

social, 1, 42, 51, 52, 67, 69, 83, 87, 96, 112

soft drink, 49, 50, 62, 86

stillbirth, 13, 54, 89

stress, 5, 6, 7, 15, 26, 34, 49, 51, 59, 60, 62, 70, 101, 104, 106, 107, 108, 110, 111, 112, 122, 123, 128

sugar-sweetened drink, 10

sweets, 49, 50, 61, 62

synapse, 4, 70, 79, 99

third trimester, 4, 20, 22, 30, 56, 105, 108, 120

tofu, 40, 72

twin, 17, 57

underweight, 12, 24, 25, 57

vegetable, 10, 15, 28, 31, 33, 34, 36, 37, 39, 63, 72, 116, 118

vegetarian, 29, 74

vitamin A, 47, 76

vitamin D, 41, 42, 47, 58, 73, 74

weight gain, 25, 50, 56, 57, 58, 59, 63, 110

working memory, 26, 51, 87

yogurt, 31, 47, 48, 61

ABOUT THE AUTHOR

Chong Chen is a research scientist at the RIKEN Brain Science Institute in Wako, a suburb of Tokyo, Japan. He studied at Hokkaido University, where he obtained a Ph.D. in Medicine and won several academic awards, including the Takakuwa Eimatsu Award.

Chong has been the author of some 20 articles, all of which have been published in professional journals and which cover several aspects of his fields of expertise; neuroscience, psychiatry and psychology.

In addition to these important pieces, Chong has written two books. *Fitness Powered Brains: Optimize Your Productivity, Leadership and Performance*, is exactly what it sounds like and is ideal for business people, while *Plato's Insight: How Physical Exercise Boosts Mental Excellence* shows how being physically active can directly correlate to mental ability and how this fact has been known for centuries. In fact, one of Plato's quotations was part of the inspiration for the title – "with education and exercise, man can attain perfection."

When he has free time, Chong likes to get some fresh air and exercise by cycling. He also loves playing ping-pong, reads novels and poems and is a huge fan of the Argentine Tango.

As far as the future goes, Chong hopes that he will be able to translate scientific findings into ways that will allow regular people to live better lives. And through his books, he hopes that he can reach a much wider audience.

You can contact Chong Chen and follow what he is writing about at:

https://brainandlife.net

Twitter: @ChongChenBlog

Email: chen@brainandlife.net